THE LONGEVITY DIET PLAN

The Beginner's Guide To Weight Loss, Reduce Inflammation and Heal The Immune System with healthy lifestyle

By Michael Clark

Text Copyright ©

Legal & Disclaimer

BOOK1

CHAPTER 13: HEALTHY AND DELICIOUS BEVERAGES

BOOK2

Anti-inflammatory diet

A comprehensive guide for the Anti-inflammatory diet plan

Book Description

Inflammation can hijack our feelings of wellness and slow us down, but when it becomes chronic, this may signal that something is out of alignment in our diet or lifestyle. Normal inflammation occurs in the body on a regular basis as part of our natural process of maintaining a healthy internal balance. It's only when the necessary process of inflammation gets out of hand that well-being can become impaired.

We'll also present the principles of an easy anti-inflammatory diet, based on whole foods and grounded in science, to support you in restoring your natural balance. Our simple lists of foods to include (and those to avoid) will help you choose meals far beyond the recipes. We'll also touch on how people's bodies respond differently to particular ingredients, so you can personalize these recipes to best meet your own nutritional needs.

The more difficult side of this equation is that the visceral fat is not one that ever truly leaves the body. It is the fat that hides out in all of the nooks and crannies of your abdominal organs, which makes it dangerous to remove with such invasive procedures as liposuction. Neither will these fat cells dissipate from your body with weight loss and exercise. However, as you reduce obesity levels, these fat cells respond by reducing in size, and that reduction slows down the production of as many harmful, inflammatory chemicals.

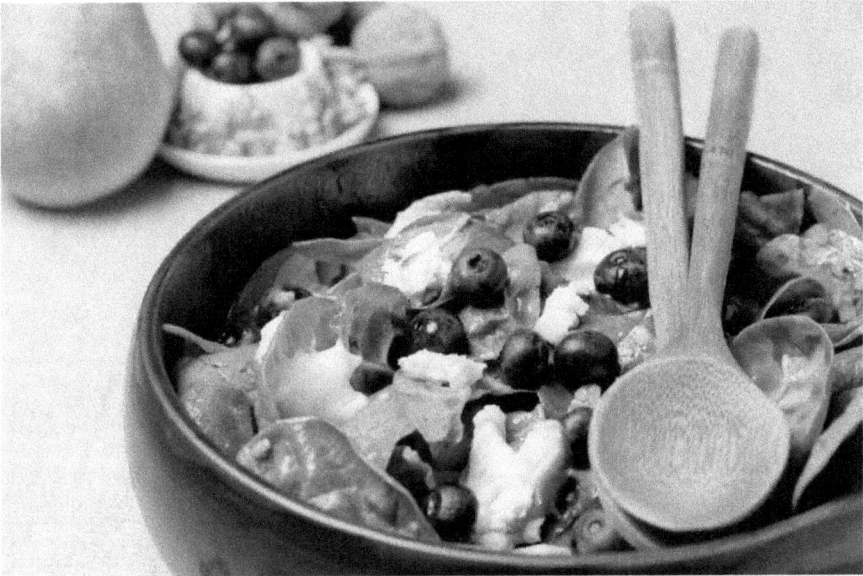

INTRODUCTION

A good and healthy diet can do miracles no medicine in this world can do. With a good diet, you can ensure a disease-free life with active metabolism. Our body goes through a constant process of self-repairment and experiences various phenomenon on the way.

Inflammations are therefore a temporary process of regeneration and reintegration of normal conditions following a damage; however, if the harmful agents persist or if there is a production of mainly type 1 cytokines, it can become chronic. In this case one can observe a progressive reduction of the microcirculation processes described above - as it happens during the recovery - while at the same time the infiltrated cells are progressively constituted by macrophages and lymphocytes that are frequently disposed around the vascular wall like a sleeve, which causes its compression. As a consequence, a state of tissue suffering is established, which is established by the presence of the infiltrate and by the reduction of blood flow caused by the vascular compression.

Inflammation is one of the body's responses to a number of environmental factors. The idea behind the conception of this book is to provide you with all the pros of opting a dietary approach to reduce or

eliminate risks of inflammation and to make you
aware of the relevant recipes. Let's get started!

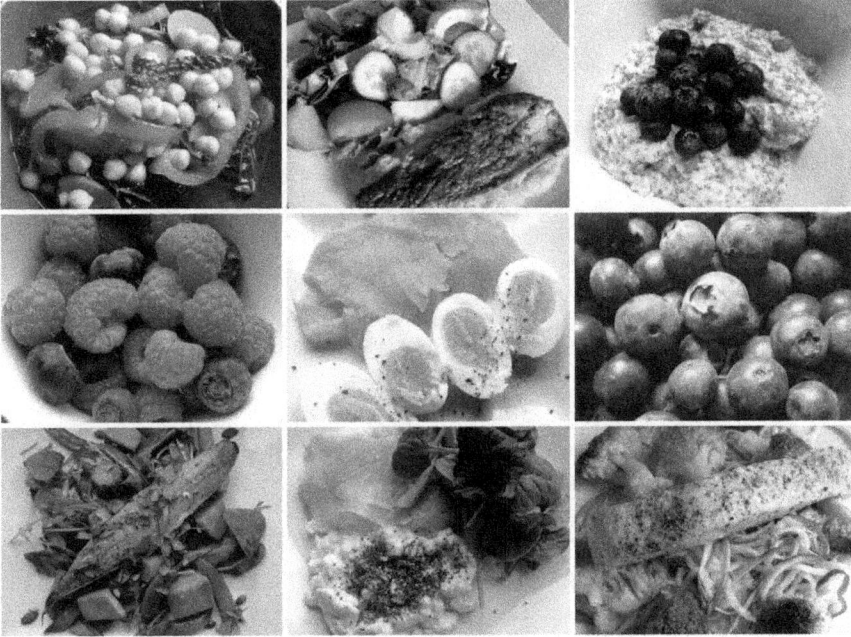

Chapter 1: What is Inflammation?

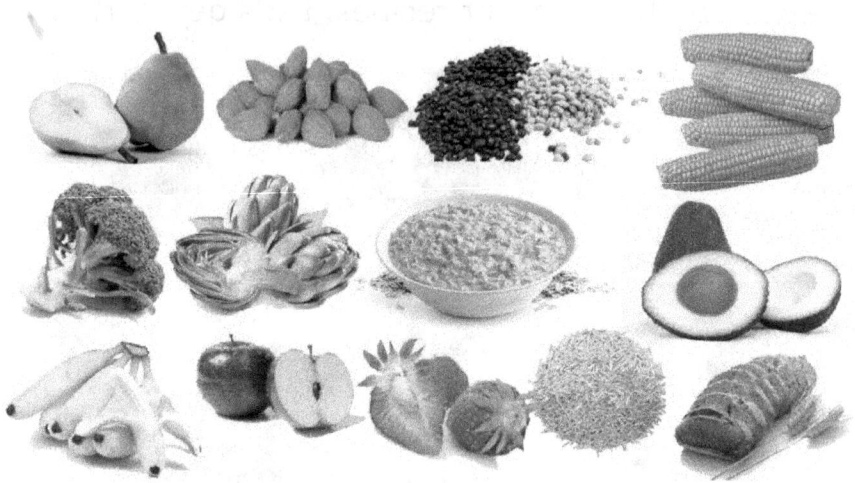

When using the terms inflammation or phlogosis one intends the set of alterations that occur in an area of the organism that has been hit by a damage of an intensity that has not affected the vitality of all cells within the area. Such damage could be induced by physical agents (such as traumas or heat), chemical agents (such as toxic components or acids) and biological agents (such as bacteria and viruses).

The response to the damage, the inflammation in fact, is given by the cells that have survived it and is therefore primarily a local reaction. Medical terminology defines the reaction by adding -tis to the name of the organ that is inflamed (for example the terms tendinitis and hepatitis indicate, respectively, a tendon and liver inflammation). The reaction was defined as primarily local instead of exclusively local as several molecules that are synthesized and released by the cells that participate in the phenomenon move into the blood and operate on long distanced organs, especially the liver. Thus, stimulating the liver cells to release other substances that are responsible for the acute response phase to the inflammation. The presence of a fever and leucorrhoea (which is an increase in the number of leukocytes circulating in the blood) represent other systematic indications of phlogosis. The inflammation itself is a useful process to the organism, as it allows it to neutralize (if present) the agent that has caused damage, and reintegrate the normal condition pre-existing to the detrimental event.

In the case of muscular injury, for example, the inflammation process that follows is especially necessary to activate a subdivided process of the very own damage (in this case the agent generating the damage would be a physical agent, like a trauma, and there will be no necessity to eliminate the damaging agent, unlike in other cases).

The most known symptoms of inflammations are an increase in the local temperature, swelling, redness, soreness, and functional compromission. The phenomenons that cause such symptoms are mainly caused by events that involve the microcirculation of blood. An extremely rapid vasoconstriction is followed by the relaxation of the smooth muscular fiber cells present on terminal arterioles' walls, with resulting vasodilation and increasing blood flow to the traumatized area (which causes the increase in local temperature and redness). Subsequently, the higher blood flow stagnates in the traumatized zone, thus increasing the blood's viscosity (given by the red blood cells' aggregation and by the plasma's outflow to the intercellular junctions); leukocytes will also start flowing out the blood at the extravascular compartment where they are attracted by specific cytokines. Thus, the exudate is formed, which is the root of the swelling. It is constituted partly by a liquid and partly by suspended cells in it. Finally, the subdivided process of cellular damage will start.

The set of processes that is described above is mediated by various molecules which trigger, maintain and also limit the modifications in the microcirculation. Such molecules are called chemical mediators of phlogosis, and they can come from different sources and have different scopes. These are histamine, serotonin, arachidonic acid's metabolites (prostaglandines, leukotrienes and thromboxanes), lysosomal enzymes, type 1 and type 2 cytokines, nitric oxide, the kinin system and the complement system. Instead, the cells that intervene in the inflammatory processes are constituted by mastocytes, basophils, neutrophils and eosinophils, monocytes/macrophages, natural killer cells, platelets, lymphocytes, plasma cells, endothelial cells and fibroblasts.

Next, fibroblasts can be stimulated to proliferate, with the consequence that many chronic phlogosis cases culminate with an excessive formation of connective tissue which constitutes fibrosis or sclerosis. For example, that is the case for cellulite, a socially unaesthetic disease which affects many women, caused by the increase in volume of adipose cells in some areas of the body (mostly thighs and glutes) with the lack of liquid draining and the process of local inflammation which can induce, at the worst phases, fibrosis and sclerosis with the formation of micronodules which give skin the classic "orange peel" aspect.

The inflammation itself can therefore be defined as a "physiologic" response of the organism to a detrimental stimulus (for example a cut or a trauma) and it can be of the acute kind (angio phlogosis), mainly involving the modifications to the vascular system to ease the reparation of the damage and the inflow of the immune system cells, or it can be chronic, of long duration and with a persistent reaction by the immune system. During these processes, it was clear how chemical mediators are generated in great quantities, such as inflammatory cytokines, which not only have a local action in the damaged tissue but also flow throughout the whole body and "inflame" it in chronic conditions.

That is the case, for example, for the pathological alterations of the Intestinal Microbiome (see related chapter) or more generally of the intestinal barrier with the diffusion of material from the enteric lumen in the blood flow and generation of a low level chronic inflammatory state.

Over time such conditions can increase the risk of many metabolic pathologies like obesity, diabetes mellitus and metabolic syndrome. Here is why it is good to know how to "deinflammate" our organism also through our diet choices.

Chapter 2: T of Inflammation?

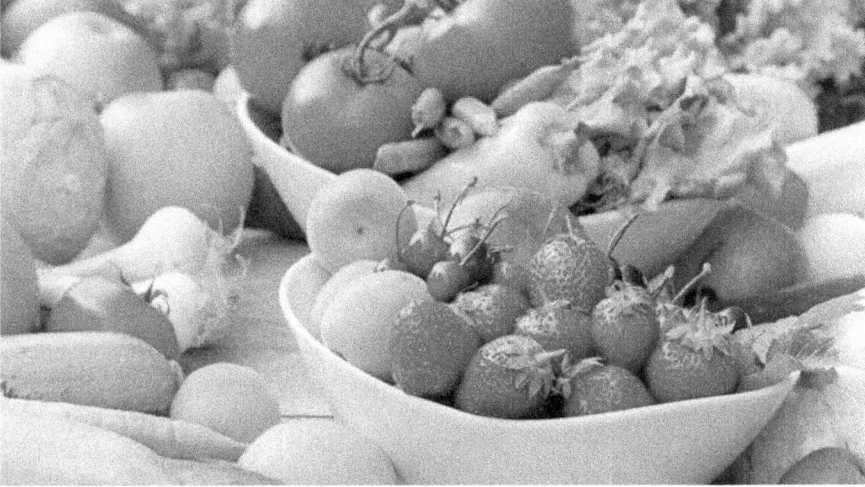

You should know the two major types of inflammation to better deal with it. These are:

Acute inflammation:

It is the instantaneous response of the body in the result of damage to body cells. Swelling occurs within 2 to 3 seconds of the injury. It doesn't persist for a longer duration.

Acute inflammation is one that starts quickly and becomes serious in a brief time. Signs or symptoms are normally just present for a couple of days and nights but may persist for a couple of weeks in some instances.

Systemic or Chronic inflammation:

It is a long-term inflammation, which is often caused due to allergies, cancer, diabetes, lungs diseases, asthma, heart complexities, etc. In these cases, the inflammation is cured only by treating the root cause.

Inflammation may be the defense reply that centers your immune system's consideration toward combating a perceived menace -- often microorganisms or Trojans or harm from international invaders, like poisons. When a section of your body becomes reddened, swollen, very hot and often agonizing, this is swelling in action.

Great up to now. But when swelling is chronically fired up, the immune system's capability to fight off different insects and pathogens will be compromised.

Chronic inflammation is frequently regarded as the effect of your "overactive" disease fighting capability -- as if your immune purpose is perplexed or malfunctioning. But can be this definitely what's going on? Or carry out we just reside in an increasingly harmful and stressful entire world?

After all, a lot of people today are confused with anxiety and environmental poisons, like endocrine-disrupting and cancer-causing substances from food to drinking water to household cleansers. And your body has every right to respond defensively. Foods allergies, poor diet program, toxins, and pressure are the most important culprits.

To combat irritation, we have to help our anatomies deal with this continuous harm of immune causes. One of the better ways to aid your body in combatting inflammation would be to consume an anti-inflammatory diet program.

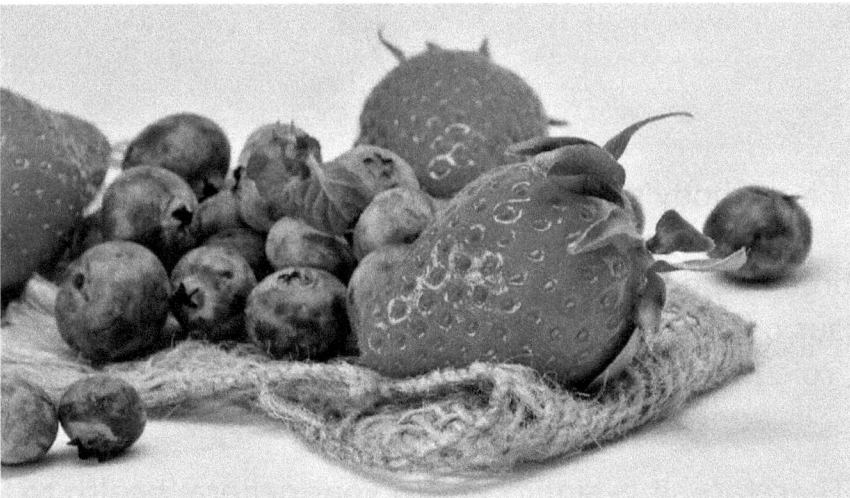

Chapter 3: Myths, misconceptions and mistakes made by individuals

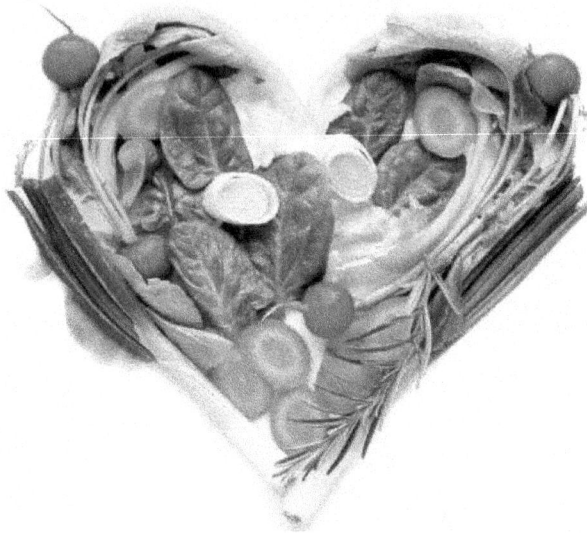

Your body's metabolism dictates your ability to produce energy. Metabolism is the process of breaking down food particles by the organic cells of your body. The metabolic process also plays a crucial role in your ability to burn fat to attain your ideal body weight.

Therefore, it is significant to your general health to have a high capacity of burning fat for energy. In short, it is always paramount to enhance your body's metabolic process.

Repeatedly, people are engaging in activities and behaviors. that are wrecking their metabolism.

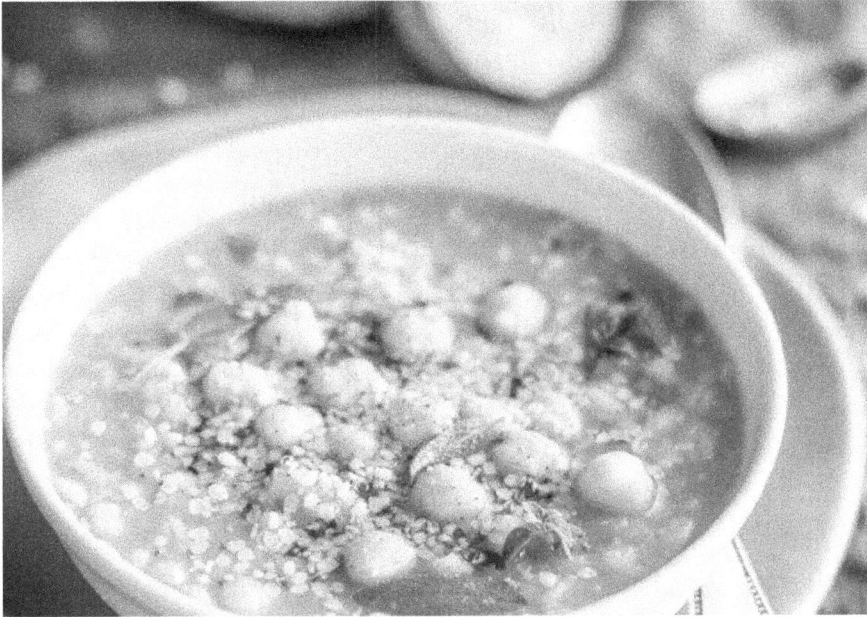

Worse, they are unaware of it all! The anti-inflammatory diet directly refers to the metabolic processes and the immune system of your body. Hence, therein gushes forth most of the common mistakes, misunderstandings, and misconceptions of practicing the regimen.

Here is a compilation of the top mistakes while practicing the regimen. Learning these common errors will help you to avoid these glitches along the way. The list also includes the corresponding tips:

Misstep #1: Concentrating on Calories & Heedless on Hormones

One of the most misinterpreted myths misguiding many people is the assumption that the weight of the body bears a direct connection to the number of calories consumed. This outdated perception is an erroneous way of looking at how your body's metabolic functions. You should instead embrace the significant reality of linking your caloric consumptions with your hormonal and body functions. The reality is that the types of food that you consume can alter your hormones completely and hinder the efficiency of your metabolism to burn fat.

In other words, consuming a calorically similar regimen of refined carbs against low-glycemic indexed whole foods will produce different effects on your metabolic processes. Likewise, indulging in a low-carb diet compared to a high-carb diet will cause advantageous outcomes on how your cells will burn fat for fuel, regardless of your caloric intake.

Again, your hormones and metabolism operate beyond food consumption. Your five primary hormones, which control your fat-burning process, are insulin, leptin, ghrelin, cortisol, and adiponectin. An array of factors influences these hormones such as your regular exercise routines, sleep quality, stress levels, hydration levels, and diet.

☐ Myth-1: Curb Carbs, Fill Fats

– Lowering your carb intakes and increasing your consumption of healthy fats makes a great difference towards improving your metabolism. Such a regimen simultaneously helps to stabilize your blood sugar levels, decreases insulin levels, and boosts the burning of fats. Consuming a surplus of carbs tends to convert the excesses into fats, stored as fatty tissues. Their regular consumption characterizes typically a chronically high blood sugar level, which results in a diverse range of destructive effects on your body.

However, switching your body into a fat-burning machine is technically engaging with a low-carb and high fat (LCHF) diet. Research supports this dietary model since it outperforms a low-fat regimen in countering obesity, diabetes, and other inflammatory factors.

☐ Myth-2: Short & Strenuous Exercise Engagements – Your exercise habits significantly contribute to the general health of your hormones.

Many people indulge in daily exercises with the aim of losing weight in the wrong way. Low-intensity cardio workouts daily are harmful to your body and as such, unnecessary.

Instead, short-duration and high-intensity intermittent exercises (HIIE) are highly effective for hormone enhancement. Modern studies confirm that these more explosive modes of exercises provide increased benefits for shedding weight as opposed to other forms of exercises.

Among the more well-known examples of these workouts are those boxing sessions or 30-second sprints followed by an active recovery activity of 2 to 4 minutes (usually, walking or other forms of low-intensity body movements). If ever you deem such exercises as severely intensive for your body, then you can always modify them.

An ideal phase, to begin with, would be 30 seconds of performing each exercise program, followed by another 30 seconds of resting. You may also Adjust the exercise movements to make them less straining or comfortably easier.

Nonetheless, your aim should be pushing yourself to your limits of performing high-intensity exercises. Attaining this objective allows your body to adapt to an appropriate hormonal balance gained from these typical exercises.

☐ Myth-3: Terminate Toxic Substances & Supplies – Accumulated toxins in your body can directly lead to poor fat metabolism. For instance, in today's modern society, many food chemical components can mimic the functions of estrogen (a hormone promoting fat retention) with potentials for completely disrupting a hormonal balance.

You can prevent exposing your body to such risks by eating only wild-caught or pasture-raised meats and organically grown vegetables. Furthermore, avoid using beauty products, synthetic plastics, unfiltered water, and other similar supplies filled with toxic substances.

Always be aware of what you introduce to your body. Check and use only products that contain natural ingredients as much as possible.

Misstep #2: Mindless on Micronutrients

For most of us, we spend the majority our time focusing more on our consumptions of fats, proteins, and carbohydrates— the major macronutrients. Although the amount of each of these macronutrients is a vital factor for healthy nutrition planning, the number of micronutrients may disputably be more significant. Your body uses dozens of various beneficial micronutrient substances.

These micronutrients include vitamins, minerals, fatty acids, enzymes, antioxidants, and all sorts of essential compounds contained in foods. Their role is to keep you energized, produce hormones and digestive enzymes, repair and rejuvenate cells and tissues, mineralize bones, slow down oxidation damage or aging caused by free radicals, and prevent nutritional deficiencies. Deficiencies of specific micronutrients may lead to various health issues such as bone loss, thyroid problems,poor digestion, and mental impairment. Notably, a low level of micronutrient consumption influences your body's metabolism directly in a manner that promotes a major gain of fats.

For instance, nutrients such as zinc, selenium, and iodine serve to produce thyroid hormones. When you severely lack these nutrients, you may incur lower thyroid hormone productions and a much slower metabolism.

☐ Myth-1: Rainbow Ration Regimen – Various colors in diverse foods represent the presence of corresponding types of nutrients and unique benefits. For instance:

☐ Red Foods – are rich in carotenoids that are beneficial for your heart, eyes, immune system, blood, joints, and skin.

☐ Orange Foods – are excellent sources of fiber and vitamin C that promote collagen growth. They also contain cryptoxanthins— antioxidants that protect cells from damage and cancer growths.

☐ Purple & Blue Foods – are high in powerful anthocyanins— antioxidants that protect against heart disease, improve mineral absorption, enhance exercise performance, boost brain function, and other highly anti-inflammatory mechanisms. Purple and blue foods can even synergize well with a high-fat regimen to accelerate fat burning.

☐ Green Foods – contain trace minerals, chlorophyll, and sets of the B-vitamins and Vitamin K that detoxify your body, fight free radicals, and improve your immune system.

In particular, green foods are leafy greens, which are ideal inclusions to low-carb nutrition that support fat metabolism.

☐ Yellow Foods – possess antioxidant compounds that convert into vitamins C, B6, and A, potassium, phosphorus, riboflavin, fiber, magnesium, and folate. All these help to improve your heart functions, vision, digestive, and immune systems.

☐ White Foods – have lots of vitamins, minerals, and other vital food nutrients that your body needs to maintain a healthy weight and to protect against various inflammatory diseases.

☐ Myth-2: Mineral Maintenance – Your body requires both major and minor trace minerals to maintain optimum wellness. These minerals are necessary for your enzymes to function appropriately apart from supporting essential metabolic processes such as thyroid hormone production.

Generally, the required amount of trace minerals for your body should be less than 100 milligrams a day.

The key trace elements are zinc, selenium, molybdenum, manganese, iron, iodine, copper, cobalt, and chromium.

They are nature's catalysts that stimulate the work of enzymes, which further generate all metabolic processes necessary for life.

Deficiencies in mineral intake disable your body to gain adequate energy, proper bone formation, blood circulation and maintain optimal levels of hormone production. Excellent sources of minerals include the following:

☐ Avocados

☐ Fermented Foods

☐ Ghee or Grass-Fed Butter

☐ Grass-Fed Meats

☐ Leafy Greens

☐ Olives

☐ Pasture-Raised Eggs

☐ Pink Salts

☐ Sea Vegetables

☐ Vegetable or Bone Broth

☐ Wild-Caught Fish

☐ Myth-3: Staple Supplements – Myopic or careless farming practices have resulted in poor soil conditions in several areas of the world. For this reason, it becomes more unreliable to determine whether farm products or the foods you eat contain proper levels of nutrients, which they should. Therefore, having a staple of daily food supplements is essential.

To cover all of your bases, an excellent strategy is to consume multi-vitamins, multi-minerals, or all-in-one superfoods. You do not necessarily need to take all these in one sitting, but consuming at least one of them is highly advisable, especially if you are nutrient-deficient.

A huge mistake most people commit is to leave their digestive problems unaddressed, particularly when trying to figure out their metabolism issues. Thus, if you are experiencing any digestive issues like leaky gut or dysbiosis (gut bacterial imbalance), reduced stomach acids, and small intestinal bacterial overgrowth (SIBO), then it is difficult for your body to regulate hunger, much less, absorb all the food nutrients.

Furthermore, your body will have a sluggish metabolism that will leave you overweight and feeling lethargic. Poor digestion may also cause an undesirable spiral of effects that stifle your metabolism and thyroid hormone conversion.

Misstep #3: Availing Needlessly Anti-Nutrients

Anti-nutrients either deplete or prevent absorption of other useful nutrients in your body. They may manifest in various forms such as the following:

☐ Toxins – heighten the demand for detoxifying the liver. The delicate detoxification process requires the involvement of various multiple nutrients. These nutrients somehow include food products that contain antibiotics, artificial sweeteners, heavy metals,herbicides, pesticides, and other chemical elements within or on them.

The most common types of these toxic anti-nutrients are non-organic foods and processed vegetable oils. Both food items highly tend to contain pesticides, which damage your gut and deplete nutrients from your body.

Processed vegetable oils do not provide your body with a source of fuel. Besides, they are highly inflammatory. The more you consume them, the more you should eat consume omega-3 fats just to offset the harmful effects.

☐ Sugars –stimulate the process of glycolysis (breaking down sugars and carbohydrates), thus causing high sugar levels in the blood. These processes deplete vitamins B, C, and D, as well as calcium, chromium, and magnesium minerals in your body.

When consumed in excess, sugars may even lead to disruptions in cellular energy production. In effect, energy deficiencies slow down the protective mechanisms of metabolism.

☐ Phytates, Lectins, and Oxalates – are plant-based anti-nutrient proteins and compounds. People are often unaware of eating them because they are essential constituents of many everyday food items.

Plants are immobile and unable to protect themselves from various predators by either a 'fight or flight' response. Instead, they create compounds— phytates, lectins, and oxalates— that are micro toxins or poisonous for their predators.

☐ Myth-1: Avoid Anti-Nutrients Necessarily – Limiting your intakes of anti-nutrients requires you to know their chief origins. For instance, phytates generally come from legumes, grains, and nuts. While phytates are healthy for your body, they constrict the absorption of minerals such as zinc, magnesium, and calcium. Oxalates are commonly present in beets, cacao, nuts, raspberries, seeds, and spinach. Lectins are predominant in nightshade vegetables, seeds, nuts, legumes, and grains.

You do not need to avoid them altogether, but it is prudent to lessen your consumptions of these plant-based anti-nutrients. Otherwise, you will eventually incur serious gut health issues, chronic pain, or kidney problems.

☐ Myth-2: Soaking & Steaming Preparation Procedures – To further augment the reduction of anti-nutrient content in some foods, you should practice soaking seeds and nuts in filtered water right on the eve before you use or consume them. Some nuts and seeds may sprout after soaking them. These processes of soaking and sprouting unveil a higher nutritional profile, making the nuts and seeds more suitable for your digestive tract.

Raw cruciferous (mustard family) of vegetables can be direct sources of anti-nutrients, which pose difficulties on your digestive tract. A better way to lessen the disabling effects of these typical vegetables is to steam them before eating. Steaming also serves to break down exterior cellulose fibers gently, and thus, making it easier for your digestive tract system to process. Fermenting is also another viable option.

Misstep #4: Treating Thirst as Hydrating Hunger

Mostly, people easily misinterpret thirst for hunger. Yet the reality is that a dehydrated body can convey a false signal to your brain, indicating a low blood sugar and prompt you to eat.

If you are engaging in a low-carb dietary plan and frequently end up feeling hungry between meals, then, you are either dehydrated or not eating enough fats. Hence, instead of grabbing immediately for a snack, drink a glass of water first and observe how you feel.

☐ Myth-1: Win Wellness with Water – Hydration is crucial on any dietary program. However, there are several recommendations for adequate water intake.

Studies note that all it takes to impair your physical performances is a water loss equivalent to 2% of your body weight. A water loss of roughly 2.8% of your body weight can reduce your cognitive functions. By these conclusions, it is vital to reiterate how your ideal water intake directly relates to your body weight.

As a basic guideline, your daily minimum water intake should be half of your total body weight (based in pounds) in ounces of water. Ideally, you should consume ¾ of your entire body weight in ounces of water per day. This recommendation is highly unlikely if you weigh more than 3,000 pounds. Nevertheless, if you are slim and lean, this advice is simple to follow as long as you stay hydrated between meals.

Applying baseline values, consider drinking more to refill the water lost from exercising. The same studies suggest that for water lost due to exercises, you should drink a half-liter (18-ounces) of water for each pound of your total body weight.

Hence, drinking water amidst your diet demands you to weigh yourself daily. This procedure allows you to know how much weight you have already lost or what weight you should ideally maintain.

Nonetheless, one of the more popular hydration strategies is to hydrate your body early in the day. For instance, drinking 1-2 liters (16-32 ounces) of water before taking your first meal is an excellent way of cleansing the body, promoting better digestion, and restoring dehydration that has just occurred overnight.

In addition, proper hydration of your body is dependent on both water and mineral contents. Combining a pinch of sea salt with your water is a bright idea to add electrolytes— body minerals found in the bloodstream, tissues, urine, and other body fluids that help to balance water retention in your body

Adding organic acids (i.e., citric and acetic acids) in your water is also a great way to improve your body's hydration and stabilize your blood sugar level. You can consume these acids in the form of lemon juice (citric acid) or apple cider vinegar (acetic acid). You only have to add a splash of either organic acids to your water to curtail your cravings until mealtime.

Chapter 4: How Dieting works

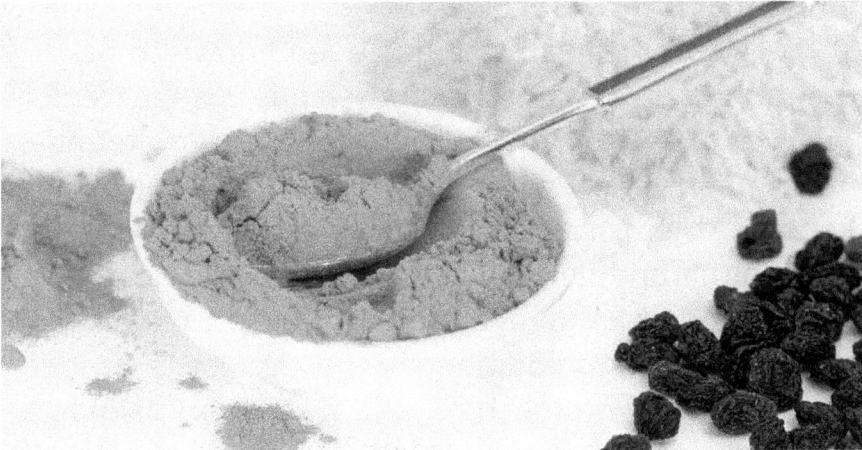

Inflammation has always been a therapeutic secret, yet now it has turned into a foe of long haul health. Additional red platelets, safe cells, and antioxidants are hurrying to the injured site to recuperate it. In any case, conveyed excessively thus far,inflammation can be lethal, as when somebody is too scorched to even consider recovering.

Just in a couple that is previous of, has it unfolded that low-level incessant inflammation, which ordinarily goes unnoticed, has an influence on numerous life disorders, for example, hypertension, heart disease, cancer, and Alzheimer's disease.

The moderate trickle, dribble of inflammatory markers, can take a very long time to make real impedance, which implies that every individual must tailor his way of life to counter them. Diet alone is not sufficient to keep ceaseless, intense inflammation under control... yet it is a decent start. The Mediterranean diet has been known to help lessen inflammation in the body, so it is an incredible way to kick-start your diet. By embracing an anti-inflammatory diet, you go for two positive outcomes: keeping the microorganisms in your digestive tracts healthy and flourishing, thereby avoiding the drainage of lethal synthetics into the circulation system. There is additionally the circuitous benefit that a healthy stomach related framework, sends a sign of prosperity along the vagus nerve to the heart and cerebrum. There is a huge number of microorganisms that possess the intestinal tract, and are a fundamental piece of our complete DNA, contributing a great many separate genomes. Together this tremendous settlement is known as the microbiome. Here are some basic focuses to know. The gut microbiome is not the same as a culture to culture.

In every one of us, it is always moves accordingly to the diet, yet to pressure and even feelings. Because of its hereditary, multifaceted nature, an "ordinary" gut microbiome has not been characterized at this point. It is accepted that flourishing, healthy gut microbiome is

established on a wide scope of common foods wealthy in fruits, vegetables, and fiber. The cutting edge Western diet, which is low in fiber, yet high in sugar, salt, fat, and handling food, might be genuinely debasing the gut microbiome. At the point when the gut microbiome is harmed or debased, microscopic organisms start to discharge supposed endotoxins— the results of microbial activity. If these poisons spill through the intestinal divider into the circulatory system, markers for inflammation are activated, and persevere until the poisons are never again present.

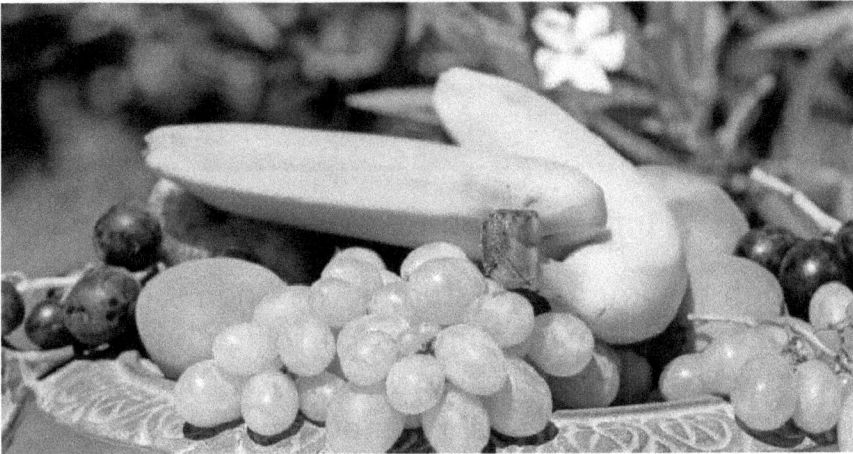

Chapter 5: An overview of Anti-Inflammatory Diet

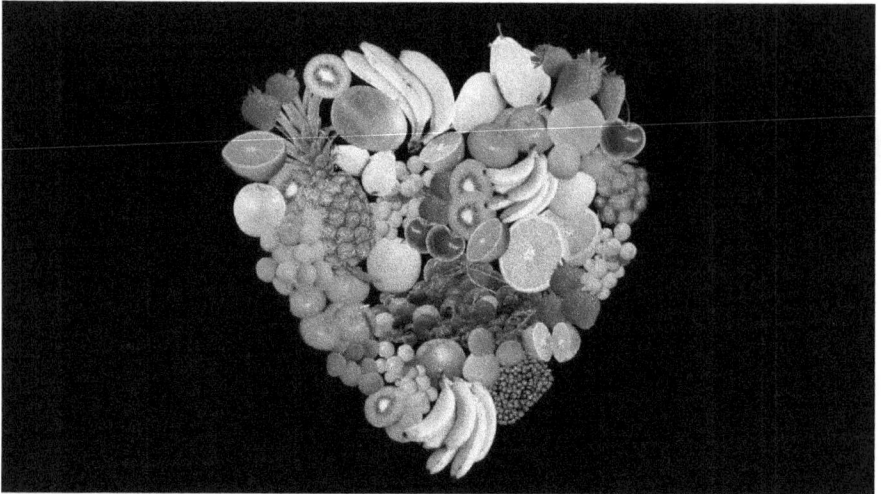

How Inflammation Helps—and Harms

When the immune system is working properly, inflammation plays an important role in our body's healthy response to injury or infection. Upon injury or infection, such as a scrape on the knee or exposure to the cold everyone else has at the office, our immune system rallies to restore health. This leads to a period of acute inflammation, which promotes healing as the body's defensive process repairs and restores integrity. Once the problem has been successfully managed, the immune response deactivates, and the inflammation around the area of injury or infection subsides.

When you notice that a paper cut on your finger is red, swollen, warm, and painful, this is all part of inflammation, which is taking place as a result of a smoothly running immune system. Immune cells have been activated to the site of the problem, so blood flow in the area increases, leading to the experience of swelling and heat, which will subside as the wound heals. Soon you'll have nothing to remember the paper cut by but a thin line of scar tissue. This kind of acute, localized inflammation may not require any additional treatment; however, maintaining a consistent anti-inflammatory diet like the one described in this book will ensure that your body has all the nutrients needed to support even this minor healing process.

Conversely, a little cut that seems to hang on too long, remaining puffy and painful and not making much progress in healing, might indicate a bigger issue. In this case, the normal process of acute inflammation may have continued unchecked, signaling a chronic inflammation that is more problematic. This can occur as a result of an unhealed infection like hepatitis B or C, prolonged exposure to environmental toxins like cigarette smoke, or existing health conditions like obesity or autoimmune disease. Lifestyle factors such as diet and stress can also amplify the inflammatory response. At first, there may not be any obvious symptoms of this kind of ongoing low-grade inflammation, yet in the long term, chronic inflammation can increase risk for or exacerbate a variety of diseases.

ANTI-INFLAMMATORY DIET GUIDELINES

Smart Dietary Choices

A whole foods approach to eating is the best route to decreasing inflammation, and that's the strategy we present here. As the benefits of anti-inflammatory diets become clearer, a growing number of studies reveal which foods are best to include or avoid as you move toward vibrant wellness. Let's check them out.

Foods That Fight Inflammation

FRUITS AND VEGETABLES. Consider yourself free to enjoy a wide range of fruits and vegetables on the anti-inflammatory diet—they're all good! Plant foods deliver a high-nutrient, low-calorie foundation and add bright, tempting color to any plate. These foods are a source of satisfying, anti-inflammatory fiber, plus vitamins, minerals, and micronutrients. Fruits and vegetables also contain powerful antioxidant compounds that help prevent cellular damage.

Berries, watermelon, apples, and pineapple in particular are proven anti-inflammatory superstars, thanks to their high levels of phytonutrients. Thousands of these chemicals can be found in different combinations in plant foods, and while they protect the plant against environmental damage, they also protect you on a cellular level, especially when you eat a wide range of produce. Citrus fruits provide high-antioxidant vitamin C, a knockout inflammation fighter. Vegetables such as onions, broccoli, and leafy greens support resistance to inflammation. Garlic and onion don't just add pungent flavor—they've also been studied extensively for their immune system benefits.

NIGHTSHADES. Beware the boundless Internet (mis)information available—some is inaccurate and not well grounded in science. Rumors that you can't enjoy nightshades such as tomatoes, potatoes, bell peppers, and eggplant on an anti-inflammatory diet are unfounded for most people. While some with autoimmune conditions like rheumatoid arthritis choose to avoid these nutritious vegetables, the Arthritis Foundation notes that no scientific data supports this, and in fact, the group cites research that shows that consumption of yellow and purple potatoes may actually lower inflammation. However, you are the expert of your own body. If you find that this restriction is supportive of your own health and well-being, then just try to include a wide range of other vegetables to ensure you are providing all the nutrition your body needs to heal. For most people, nightshade vegetables are part of a nutritious, anti-inflammatory diet. For instance, compounds such as the lycopene provided by cooked tomatoes make these vegetables standouts for fighting inflammation.

WHOLE AND ANCIENT GRAINS. Whole and ancient grains don't merely replace refined grains. They provide exciting flavors and textures, along with fiber, micronutrients, antioxidants, and protein. Naturally gluten-free grains, such as quinoa and amaranth, keep meals interesting and can be enjoyed by everyone.

GOOD FATS. We have learned that it's more important to enjoy the right kinds of fats in moderation than to try to eliminate fat altogether. Olive oil is a rich source of polyphenols, which are compounds shown to reduce indicators of inflammation, and it should be your primary cooking oil. Specialty oils like walnut oil or pumpkin seed oil add rich flavor and beneficial unsaturated fats. And we're happy to promote the benefits of dark chocolate, a delicious source of protective polyphenols—and a fine end to a meal!

OMEGA-3 FATTY ACIDS ARE ALL-STAR ANTI-INFLAMMATORY FATS. Include foods with this type of unsaturated fat frequently to optimize your whole diet approach. Fatty fish like salmon and sardines are excellent sources, as are some plant foods such as walnuts and flaxseed. Flaxseed may sound foreign, but it's been around for thousands of years, just now gaining popularity for its abundant fiber, protein, and powerful antioxidants called lignans. Consumption of flaxseed protects against inflammation and some cancers, but go for the ground version, so your body can absorb all that goodness. Seeds like hemp and chia are similarly helpful, as are pine nuts, which are actually nutrient-dense seeds.

HERBS AND SPICES. With countless options, each herb and spice has a unique profile of antioxidants and bright flavors to complement all kinds of cuisine. Turmeric deserves special mention for its proven anti-inflammatory and neuroprotective properties. Ginger, saffron, and cinnamon are other potent flavor enhancers worth trying. Herbs such as basil, rosemary, and thyme all have inflammation-fighting compounds, and their aroma and taste elevate the meal experience.

PROBIOTICS AND PREBIOTICS. What are these, anyway? Probiotics and prebiotics support immune and digestive health. Fermented foods such as yogurt, sauerkraut, pickles, tempeh, and kimchi are known as probiotic foods because they provide a direct infusion of healthy bacteria to your system in addition to their characteristic tang. Prebiotics are foods that feed those good gut bacteria—sources include high-fiber vegetables, whole grains, and beans. Cooked beans like black beans, chickpeas, and lentils also double as lean, plant-based proteins.

HEALTHY DRINKS. Washing foods down with kombucha keeps the probiotic theme going, although not everyone appreciates the sour taste of this fermented beverage! Thankfully, unsweetened teas are good beverage options—green tea is a particularly robust source of antioxidants. Drip coffee provides fiber and is one of the biggest contributors of antioxidants to the American diet—just try to keep it sugar-free. A glass of red wine from time to time provides protective resveratrol. Water is always a great choice for hydration and promotes the body's ability to detoxify at the cellular level.

OWN YOUR WATER

Water can be the most refreshing treat when you're parched. A decanter of water with sliced cucumber in a hotel lobby is a welcome sight to weary travelers. Yet it's amazing to see how many people have a hard time taking in enough water each day. If you're one of them, consider adding some fruits or herbs to your water to boost the flavor and the benefits. Buy a pretty glass pitcher; it will make the water look especially inviting. Ginger, thyme, basil, and rosemary make good herbal anti-inflammatory add-ins; beneficial fruits include orange, grapefruit, lemon, lime, apples, watermelon, and pineapple. Try water infused with blueberries and lemon, cucumber and mint, or beets and rosemary—or come up with your own favorite flavor combinations!

Foods That Worsen Inflammation

PROCESSED FOODS. There is no shortage of delicious, nourishing food to enjoy on your anti-inflammatory diet. To maximize the benefits, you'll want to leave behind those highly processed, packaged foods, as they are typically full of proinflammatory sodium, saturated fats, added sugars, and refined grains such as white flour or white rice.

AVOID ADDED SUGARS AND REFINED GRAINS FROM ANY SOURCE. These proinflammatory foods dramatically increase blood sugar, have more calories than they do nutrition, and are linked to many negative health effects.

PROCESSED AND RED MEAT. Some meats, such as ham and many deli meats, are highly processed and contain undesirable saturated fat and sodium. Red meat is another food to choose less frequently. Even lean cuts are likely to have high levels of proinflammatory saturated fats. You might be surprised to know that you should save backyard cookouts for special occasions. This is because fatty proteins like beef prepared with high-heat dry cooking methods increase production of proinflammatory substances called advanced glycation end products, or AGEs. Consider using lower-heat, moist cooking methods, such as stewing, sautéing, or poaching, to minimize this effect. Select lean, grass-fed beef options that offer protective omega-3s, in contrast with regular beef, which is high in proinflammatory omega-6 fats.

Foods to Consider with Care

Many foods fall in the middle of the health spectrum—these foods are neither the foundation of an anti-inflammatory diet nor the worst choices. These should be considered with care, depending on your own goals and current health condition. These foods are used sparingly in our recipes, and when we do include them, we offer substitutions.

CERTAIN OILS. A few plant-based oils should be approached thoughtfully. Corn, safflower, sunflower, and soy oils are high in proinflammatory omega-6s. Despite the trendiness of coconut oil on websites that promise "magic results" from consuming it in high amounts, it is a highly saturated fat, and there is no reason to believe it is healthy to consume in excess. Occasional dishes can be prepared with coconut oil, but keep olive oil as your go-to kitchen staple.

SKIN-ON DARK-MEAT POULTRY AND PORK. Skinless white-meat poultry can serve as a good source of protein. However, higher-fat dark meat and poultry with skin-on are less healthful. Many pork products contain too much fat and sodium to belong in an anti-inflammatory diet, but very lean pork, such as pork tenderloin, can be enjoyed occasionally.

NATURAL SUGARS. We all deserve a treat, and nobody wants to feel deprived. When your sweet tooth does strike, the best sweets to choose, in moderation, are natural sugars such as honey, maple syrup, and molasses rather than refined sugar products. These offer some trace micronutrients, along with the sweet taste we crave.

Unique Bodies, Unique Reactions to Food

We also treat the "Big 8" food allergens (fish, shellfish, peanuts, tree nuts, wheat, soy, eggs, and dairy) as "Consider with Care" foods, to highlight them for those individuals who need to make substitutions. Food allergies are immune system responses in which the body mistakenly responds to proteins, in otherwise wholesome foods, as a threat. Food allergies can be life threatening, and those with food allergies know they must be vigilant to ensure they are not accidentally consuming foods that will stimulate a negative immune response.

Some people have sensitivities and intolerances to particular foods that are not technically allergies, as they do not involve the immune system. The research into this area is growing but still inconclusive; for many individuals, the best barometer for food tolerance comes from simply paying attention to how you feel after consuming that food. You know your own body best, so please modify the diet we present here to your needs. If you are uncertain about how well a particular food fits into your own dietary pattern, keep note of how you react when you eat that food, and consider consulting with a registered dietitian.

For those who can consume fish and shellfish, these are potent inflammation fighters. Deep-water fish offer unparalleled amounts of omega-3 fats in a form that is very easy for the body to use in fighting inflammation, so salmon and herring can be regular staples of your diet if you are not allergic.

Peanuts and tree nuts (walnuts, cashews, etc.) are anti-inflammatory powerhouses. If you're able to eat them, small portions of almonds or pecans provide the antioxidant vitamin E, healthy fats, and a bit of protein in addition to their rich, satisfying crunch.

Most people can consume nutritious ancient grains with no problems. If you have celiac disease or are intolerant or allergic to gluten, you'll want to avoid wheat berries and barley. Ancient grains may be avoided on strict elimination diets, which are not necessary for most people wanting to reduce inflammation. We also list the more processed whole-grain products under "Consider with Care." Whole-wheat bread is a step in the right direction from white bread, but it is still highly processed.

Intact whole grains such as quinoa reign supreme for their anti-inflammatory power.

Soy is a major allergen but also a powerful inflammation fighter. Despite widespread myths, research shows that soy reduces inflammation and cancer risks for most people—great news if you enjoy popping steamed edamame in your mouth at your favorite sushi restaurant! Soy is a high-protein source of fiber, so unless you have an allergy, freely include edamame and tofu in your diet.

Eggs offer micronutrients such as choline and lutein, but they're another common allergen. While they do not appear to have specifically anti-inflammatory properties, they can serve as a good protein source in a healthy, balanced diet. If you can, consider including eggs as part of your overall dietary strategy.

Dairy is another major food allergen. Low- or non-fat dairy products, and those cultured to provide probiotics, like yogurt and kefir, should be considered with care. There is controversy over the benefits of including full-fat dairy in one's diet, but in relation to inflammation, the picture is clearer. Sources of saturated fat, like butter and cream, are best limited on an anti-inflammatory diet, so we don't use them here.

Anti-Inflammatory Food Lists

Foods in the "Enjoy" section can be eaten freely by most people. Challenge yourself to try them all! "Consider with Care" foods are nutritious for many people to consume as part of an otherwise balanced meal pattern. If you have a food allergy or other health consideration, choose one of the other options provided. The "Avoid" foods promote inflammation and can derail your efforts. Look for ways to swap those out for foods on the "Enjoy" list!

Benefits You'll See

Change can be hard—even positive change! As you begin this diet, you may find yourself challenged as you begin thinking about your meal choices in unfamiliar ways. That's a great reason to use the shopping lists and meal plans as we've presented them. This will take the guesswork and decision making out of the early stages of your transition to an anti-inflammatory lifestyle. Then you'll build confidence to begin testing out variations that work for you.

At first, you will notice that you are satisfied after each meal or snack, and that the energy you feel is more lasting throughout your day. You may find yourself getting hungry less often; this is because you're consuming more nutrient-dense foods. You may even see your skin clearing up as you remove highly processed foods and added sugars and replace them with more nourishing options that support health at the cellular level. Many people who shift to this eating style report gradual weight loss over time, which is also beneficial for reducing inflammation.

Less visible but equally important are the longer-term improvements you may notice in your health. If you happen to get a blood test from your doctor, you'll probably see the markers of inflammation, such as C-reactive protein (CRP) and interleukin 6 (IL-6), going down, and a more healthy lipid profile— higher HDL ("good") cholesterol and lower LDL ("bad") cholesterol—emerging over time. Your energy will likely be increasingly vibrant yet grounded and calm, and your body will be better able to fight off infection, whether that means just a little cold or a more significant threat. Your energy will increase, you will be better equipped to manage stress, and you'll just feel better—all qualities that can't be quantified in a lab test. Rather, you'll notice it when you bound out of bed in the morning, feeling great and ready to tackle the day—after a nourishing and satisfying anti-inflammatory breakfast, that is!

FOODS TO ENJOY

VEGETABLES (FRESH, FROZEN, OR CANNED WITHOUT ADDED SODIUM)

Alliums

Chives

Garlic*

Leeks

Onions*

Scallions

Shallots

Cruciferous Vegetables*

Arugula

Bok choy

Broccoli

Brussels sprouts

Cabbage

Cauliflower

Collard greens

Kale

Kohlrabi

Mizuna

Mustard greens

Radish greens

Romanesco broccoli/Roman cauliflower

Turnip greens

Dark Green Leafy Vegetables

Lettuces, especially romaine*

Spinach*

Swiss chard*

Root Vegetables

Beets

Carrots

Celery root/celeriac

Radishes

Rutabagas

Sweet potatoes

Turnips

Winter squash

Other Vegetables

Asparagus

Bell peppers

Corn

Fermented, probiotic vegetables*

Green beans

Mushrooms

FRUIT (FRESH, FROZEN, OR CANNED WITHOUT ADDED SUGAR)

Apples

Apricots

Avocados

Bananas

Berries*

Citrus*

Cranberries

Figs

Grapes

Kiwi

Mangos

Melons

Pineapple*

Stone fruit

FATS AND OILS

Nut oils

Olive oil*

Seed oils

WHOLE AND ANCIENT GRAINS

Amaranth*

Brown rice

Buckwheat

Millet

Oatmeal*

Popcorn

Quinoa*

Teff*

SEEDS

Chia

Flaxseed*

Hemp

Mustard

Poppy

Pumpkin

Sesame

Sunflower

HERBS AND SPICES

Basil

Bay leaf

Cilantro

Cinnamon*

Clove

Dill

Ginger*

Mint

Nutmeg

Oregano*

Paprika

Parsley

Pepper

Rosemary*

Saffron*

Sage

Tarragon

Thyme

Turmeric*

PROTEINS

Beans*

Tempeh*

Tofu

OTHER

Unsweetened coffee

Unsweetened black or green tea*

Note: Asterisks indicate foods that are particularly beneficial anti-inflammatory superstars.

CONSIDER WITH CARE

FATS AND OILS

Coconut

Corn

Safflower

Sesame

Soy

Sunflower

WHOLE AND ANCIENT GRAINS

Barley

Emmer

Farro

Rye

Spelt

Wheat berries

Whole-grain breads, bulgur, couscous, pastas

NUTS AND SEEDS

Peanuts

Tree nuts* (e.g., almonds, cashews, macadamias, pistachios, walnuts*)

DAIRY

Fermented, probiotic dairy* (e.g., kefir, yogurt)

Low-fat and non-fat dairy products (e.g., cheese, milk)

PROTEINS

Eggs

Fish* (e.g., cod, flounder, halibut, mackerel, salmon,* sardines,* tuna)

Pork (very lean cuts, such as pork tenderloin)

Poultry (skinless white meat)

Shellfish (e.g., mussels, oysters, scallops)

Soy (e.g., edamame/soybeans, tofu, tempeh)

OTHER

Dark chocolate

Red wine

AVOID

FATS AND OILS

Butter

Lard

Margarine

GRAINS

All refined grains (e.g., white bread and rolls, white pasta, white rice)

Packaged, processed grain-based snacks and desserts (e.g., biscuits, cakes, cereals, cookies, crackers, muffins)

Pastries

OTHER

Bacon

Beef (especially high-fat cuts, beef charred on the grill, and corn-fed beef—typically any that is not grass-fed)

Full-fat dairy (e.g., butter, cheese, cream, half-and-half, ice cream)

High-fat foods (especially those with high saturated fats or trans fats)

High-sodium foods

Packaged and processed foods

Packaged, processed meat alternatives (e.g., "garden burgers," faux chicken)

Refined added sugars (brown sugar, confectioners' sugar, high-fructose corn syrup, white sugar)

73

Chapter 6: Weight Loss and the Importance of Calories

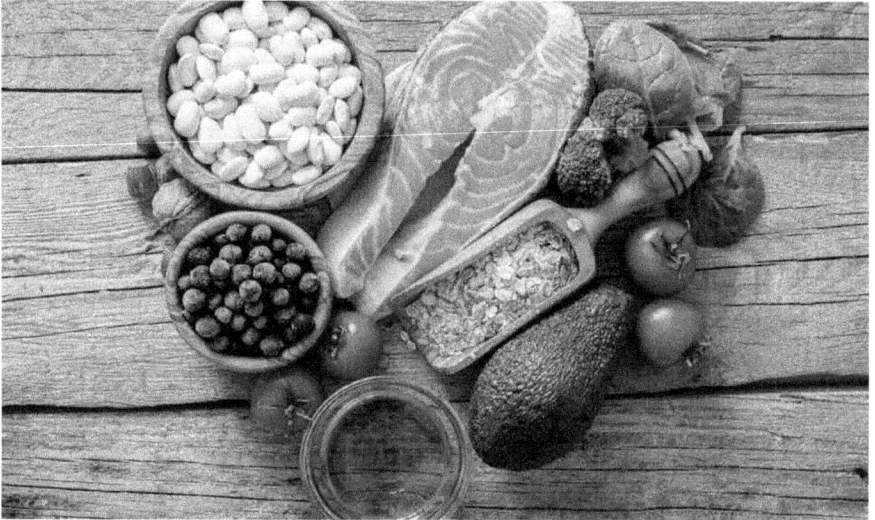

Obesity is one of these, especially if you have one of those "apple-shaped" body types where you are thicker around the middle. As previously noted, the visceral belly fat that hangs out among the organs of your abdomen does produce more of the markers in your blood stream that tell your physician that you are suffering from inflammation. The more of this "belly fat" that can be reduced, the better control you have over the reduction of those produced chemicals that aid in the development and flare ups of inflammation.

Lose Weight and Feel Great with the Anti-Inflammatory Diet

By slimming down, diminishing the amount of body fat you hold all together, you will begin to decrease the size of those visceral fat cells. The nice, added benefits include a weight loss that helps decrease or eliminate extra pressure on our joints and organs, in turn helping to alleviate some of the pain initially compounded by the inflammation.

One example that helps to explain this is the ratio of pounds to pressure on the knees. One extra pound of weight on your body exerts four extra pounds of pressure on your knees. It is how the body is built to distribute the weight. This means that by losing only ten pounds, you will reduce the amount of pressure on your knees by forty pounds!

Consider how it feels lifting forty pounds of groceries from the car (there are many who can't even do that much in one shot). Think about how you feel when you carry them into the house. The movement, the walking, etc. Adds that additional pressure to the joints of the knees, not to mention the arms, shoulders, and back. When they are put down, your body heaves a little sigh of relief. That extra weight pulling and pressing on our joints and muscles can hurt!

When you lose ten pounds, you are removing an extra forty pounds in just pain and pressure on the knees, let alone how it affects your other joints and muscles. Your body becomes more agreeable and maybe nags you just a little less. After all, pain is the body's way of telling you that something needs to change. It is protecting itself. You are coming to an agreement with your body that you will stop and reduce the pressure that you have been putting on it, while it, in turn, responds by agreeing to reduce the pain it has been causing with its nagging for you to take better care of it.

Let's take a look at a few other things that can help you have more agreeable communication with your body. Movement is one of these. If you are like most people, when you are in pain, or even feeling the general "ick" that comes with inflammation, the last thing you feel like is moving or doing anything that will draw your attention to the pain. And yet, what happens when you sit too long in one position and then have to get up and move anyway, for whatever reason? Your muscles and joints groan loudly in protest because they were quite comfortable with sitting still, pretending they didn't hurt in the first place. Your immediate reaction is usually one of not wanting to move because it hurts, and no one wants to hurt!

But we all do have to move at some point. When you start from a place of inaction—non-movement—your muscles and connective tissues for the joints stubbornly tighten up. It takes you a moment or more to get moving again, as you have to push past the tightness, which admittedly tends to hurt more at the beginning and then usually lessens as you keep going. By making movement a natural part of your day, you reduce the amount of stiffness that sets in, in turn reducing the amount of pain you feel when you do need to move.

Why does this happen? Besides the stiffening up and pain avoidance response, when muscles are not used, they start to weaken. When you don't continue to put weight on your bones, they lose density and weaken. The nervous system, which interacts with every part of your bodily functions, start to weaken their connection. Are you seeing a pattern here?

Healthy people who begin exercise and/or weight-lifting routines usually go through periods of muscle strain and bone ache as they begin to push their bodies to do more than they previously had. But as they push through and continue, their muscles and organs start to build up to work better together. Even the heart gets healthier as it works to keep up with the extra blood needed to be pumped to feed the level of activity that is now occurring. The capacity of the lungs increases as the demand for oxygen in the blood and to the organs increases to compensate for the healthier, growing masses of muscle and organs working together more efficiently and harmoniously. When you go to move, the body

is better prepared and doesn't give you the pain response in a protective warning.

Wouldn't it be nice to move without the anticipation of your body's bombardment of pain and protest? Of course! Unfortunately, not everyone, especially those suffering from inflammation or other reasons for long periods of inactivity, can just jump right into a strenuous regime of exercise and muscle building. If they were, they probably wouldn't be so desperately trying to find some way to reduce the pain and stress in their lives and bodies. In addition, some forms of strenuous exercise, when not properly done, can actually cause more damage to the body, and potentially increase inflammation with that damage.

Chapter 7: Planning a proper diet plan

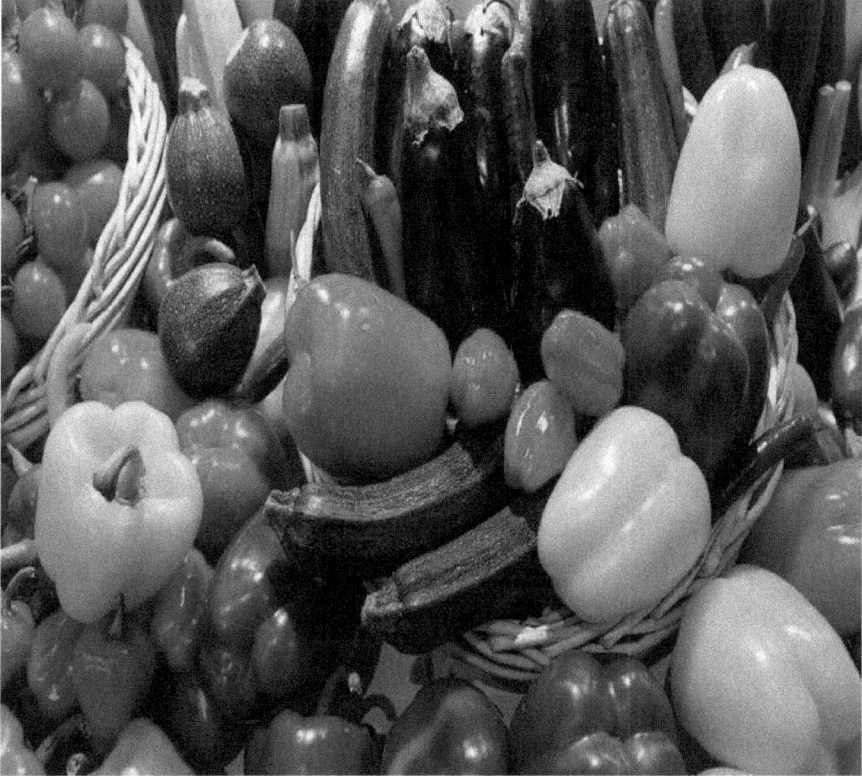

Eat more plants. Explore and enjoy the wide range of fruits and vegetables that provide fiber, antioxidants, and other nutrients to support optimal health. These low-calorie foods combat cellular damage, promote digestion, and help maintain a healthy weight range, which keeps inflammation in check as well.

Discover whole and ancient grains. Ancient grains are those that predate modern varieties created through selective breeding and hybridization—think oats, barley, chia, sorghum, quinoa, bulgur, and the like. These and whole grains retain fiber, antioxidants, and other nutrients that promote a healthy immune response. If whole grains are new to you, try mixing them 50/50 with your usual choice to begin dining the anti-inflammatory way, such as white rice with brown rice, quinoa with couscous, or whole-wheat bread crumbs with white.

Choose healthy fats. Plant-based options like olive oil contain unsaturated fats that support immunity. These are preferable to proinflammatory trans fats and saturated fats from animal products, like butter and bacon. Look for omega-3 fats, such as fish and walnuts, to directly reduce inflammation.

Enjoy nuts and seeds. These little bites provide healthy fats and protein, as well as valuable micronutrients and fiber. Plus, their flavor and crunch enhance any meal or snack.

Add flavor with herbs and spices. Turmeric, ginger, and garlic are anti-inflammatory powerhouses. Have fun exploring these and countless other options for their deep flavors and unique benefits.

Support your microbiome. High-fiber foods like beans and whole grains provide nourishment for your beneficial gut bacteria to thrive. Fermented foods such as yogurt, kimchi, and pickles keep the "communities" of bacteria in your digestive system balanced to help fight inflammation and disease.

Consume power beverages. Coffee and unsweetened black or green tea offer antioxidant compounds that promote resilience against cell damage. Enjoy red wine on occasion, if you like, to maximize anti-inflammatory benefits. Plain water is always a great choice for keeping your body hydrated and energized—vary the flavor and benefits by tossing in some cut fruit or herbs.

Eat fewer processed foods. Highly processed foods are often high in added sugars, refined grains, sodium, and detrimental fats. These types of foods are proinflammatory and also increase one's risk for weight gain and other diseases. If you haven't yet, become a label reader to increase your awareness of what's in these foods—it may surprise and inspire you to run toward the whole foods sections of the store.

Consume less meat. When you want meat, choose and prepare it carefully. Many meats have undesirable amounts of unhealthy fats, and some are pumped full of sodium during processing. Use cooking methods that do not blacken the meat, such as grilling, as the blackened parts that occur have compounds that can contribute to inflammation.

Relax! Stress is a significant contributor to inflammation and disease—in fact, chronic elevation of the stress hormone cortisol leads to ongoing negative impacts on health. Get more sleep, boost your physical activity, and try new activities such as mindfulness meditation—these all help manage stress and keep inflammation down.

Chapter 8: Balancing your Calorie intake

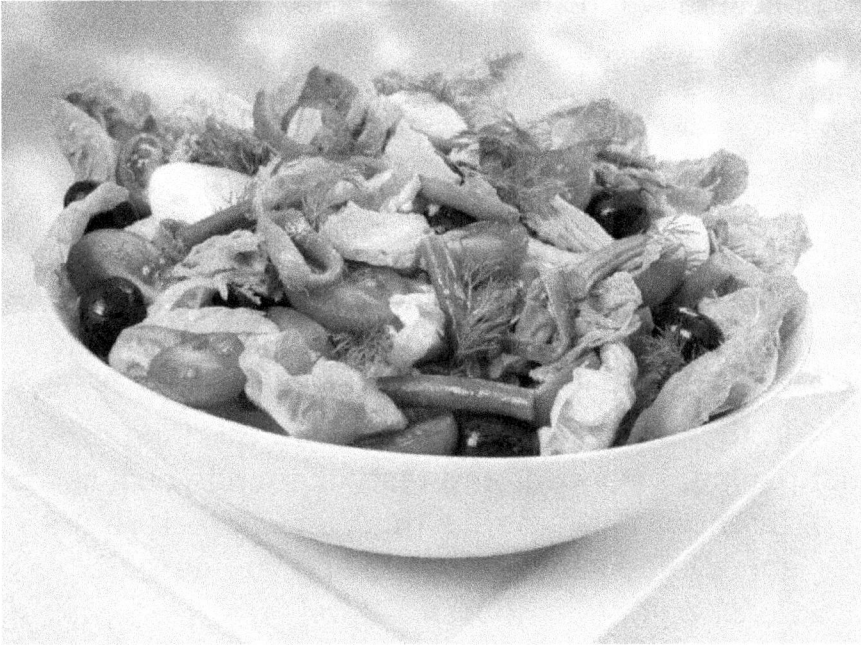

With obesity, for example, a series of causes and effects interact with each other in a downward spiral of declining health. Chronic, low-grade inflammation results directly from consumption of excess calories and obesity. As fat tissue increases, it releases chemicals, hormones, and immune cells that can disrupt normal body function. Proinflammatory cytokines are also released, leading to higher levels of inflammation throughout the body. As the internal system becomes more imbalanced, the risk of developing chronic disorders such as cardiovascular disease, hypertension, type 2 diabetes, and various cancers increases. Many of these conditions increase inflammation themselves. It can become quite complicated when so many of the body's systems are poorly regulated and caught in a feedback loop of actively causing inflammation and damage to other systems.

But there's good news! Consuming anti-inflammatory foods can help straighten out the whole situation, whatever it may be rooted in. An anti-inflammatory diet can support healing if inflammation already exists, and it will provide a foundation for resilience in the future. Shift your focus to this kind of nourishing, balanced, and tasty diet and you'll see a difference in no time, as this diet will restore the energy and sense of well-being you deserve.

Principles of the Anti-Inflammatory Diet

Experts agree that a diet consisting of a wide range of plant-based foods, accompanied by moderate amounts of whole grains, lean proteins, and healthful fats, is the type of eating pattern that will reduce inflammation and ensure a robust immune system. We are constantly learning more about the negative effects of heavily processed, packaged foods, which are often high in inflammation-promoting sodium, added sugars, refined grains, and detrimental fats. Conversely, this book emphasizes fresh, whole foods that are prepared using healthy cooking techniques. Vibrant herbs and spices are not just good for punching up flavor—you'll learn how each brings its own health-supportive qualities to your meals. Prebiotic and probiotic foods support your microbiome—that's the name for the beneficial gut bacteria in your digestive system. These bacteria are linked to a thriving immune system. And you can wash it all down with powerful inflammation-fighting beverages such as unsweetened tea and coffee, water infused with herbs or fruit, and the occasional glass of red wine, if you choose to partake.

We present recipes inspired by the many traditional cuisines around the world that promote a vigorous immune response. Traditional Japanese diets, for instance, are low in fat and full of nutrient-rich vegetables and seafood, but contain very little sugar or refined flour. A modified paleo approach is also explored here, including generous portions of vegetables and hearty protein dishes prepared from the healthiest meats. The Mediterranean eating pattern is well studied for its anti-inflammatory, health-promoting qualities, and many people find its familiar flavors satisfying and appealing. It is based on abundant fruits and vegetables, along with whole grains, legumes, and nuts. Fish, red wine, and olive oil are incorporated regularly in Mediterranean cooking, while red meat, added sugars, and high-fat dairy are limited. We are inspired by this delicious style of eating, so you'll see a lot of recipes here that reflect the Mediterranean approach. But we also recognize that the only anti-inflammatory diet that will work for you is the one you find satisfying and delicious. So after you master the basics, use these principles to figure out which styles you enjoy best and fine-tune your own anti-inflammatory lifestyle path!

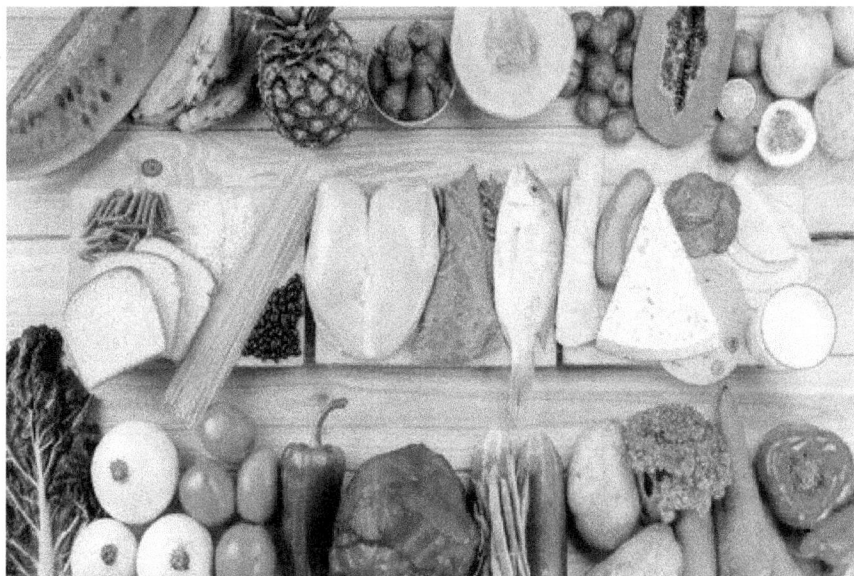

Chapter 9: Breakfast Recipes

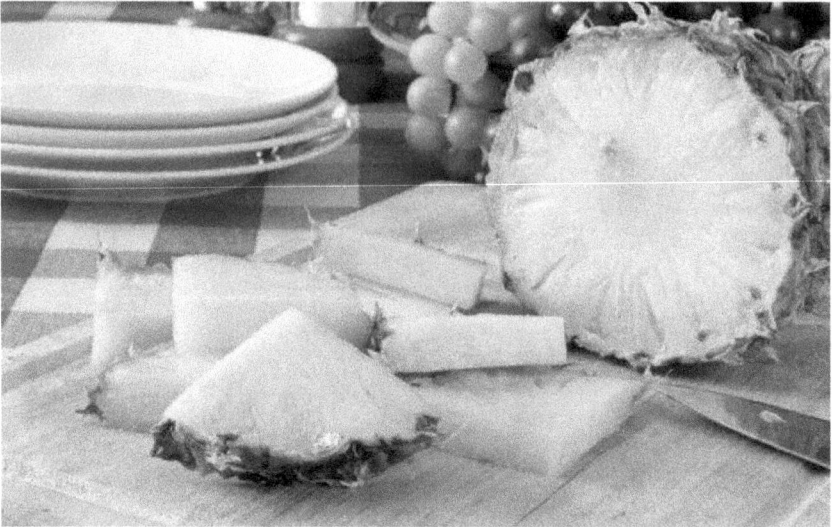

Zucchini and Sprout Breakfast Mix

Preparation time: 10 minutes

Cooking time: 0 minutes

Servings: 4

Ingredients:

2 zucchinis, spiralized

2 cups bean sprouts

4 green onions, chopped

1 red bell pepper, chopped

Juice of 1 lime

1 tablespoon olive oil

½ cup chopped cilantro

¾ cup almonds chopped

A pinch of salt and black pepper

Directions:

In a salad bowl, toss together the zucchinis with the bean sprouts, green onions, bell pepper, cilantro, almonds, salt, pepper, limejuice and oil. Serve for breakfast.

Nutrition Values: calories 140, fat 4, fiber 2, carbs 7, protein 8

Tomato and Olive Salad

Preparation time: 10 minutes

Cooking time: 0 minutes

Servings: 4

Ingredients:

2 cups baby spinach, torn

2 cups cherry tomatoes, halved

4 tablespoons chopped red onion

1 cup chopped cucumber

1 cup kalamata olives, pitted and sliced

1 tablespoon chopped dill

3 tablespoons lemon juice

A pinch of salt and black pepper

2 tablespoons olive oil

Directions:

In a salad bowl, toss the spinach with the tomatoes, onion, cucumber, olives, dill, lemon juice, salt, pepper and oil. Serve for breakfast.

Enjoy!

Nutrition Values: calories 171, fat 2, fiber 5, carbs 11, protein 5

Blueberry and Cashew Mix

Preparation time: 10 minutes

Cooking time: 12 minutes

Servings: 2

Ingredients:

2 bananas, peeled and sliced

¼ cup cashews

¼ cup blueberries

1 tablespoon almond butter

1/3 cup coconut flakes, unsweetened

1 cup coconut milk, unsweetened

Directions:

In a small pot, mix the berries with the coconut flakes, milk, cashews, almond butter and bananas. Mix together and bring to a simmer over medium heat. Cook for 12 minutes, divide into bowls and serve for breakfast.

Enjoy!

Nutrition Values: calories 370, fat 23, fiber 6, carbs 40, protein 8

Easy Almond Zucchini Bowl

Preparation time: 10 minutes

Cooking time: 15 minutes

Servings: 2

Ingredients:

1 cup egg whites, whisked

1½ tablespoons ground flaxseed

1 cup almond milk, unsweetened

1 banana, peeled and mashed

1 small zucchini, grated

½ teaspoon ground cinnamon

Directions:

In a small pan, combine the milk with the egg whites, flaxseed, banana, zucchini and cinnamon powder. Bring to a simmer, mixing constantly, over medium heat. Cook for 15 minutes, divide into bowls and serve for breakfast.

Enjoy!

Nutrition Values: calories 201, fat 6, fiber 9, carbs 14, protein 6

Sweet Potato Hash

Preparation time: 10 minutes

Cooking time: 15 minutes

Servings: 4

Ingredients:

1 sweet potato, peeled and cubed

1 celery root, peeled and cubed

1 cup coconut milk

2 tablespoons olive oil

1 small yellow onion, chopped

1 teaspoon smoked paprika

4 garlic cloves, minced

2 tablespoons parsley, chopped

A pinch of salt and black pepper

Directions:

Heat up a pan with the oil over medium-high heat. Add the celery root and the sweet potato, toss and cook for 5 minutes. Add the onion, garlic, salt, pepper, parsley and paprika then toss and cook for 8 minutes more. Add the coconut milk, mix and cook for 1-2 minutes. Divide everything into bowls and serve for breakfast.

Enjoy!

Nutrition Values: calories 188, fat 2, fiber 8, carbs 10, protein 4

Zucchini Breakfast Salad

Preparation time: 10 minutes

Cooking time: 0 minutes

Servings: 4

Ingredients:

2 zucchinis, spiralized

1   cup beets, baked, peeled and grated

½ bunch kale, chopped

2 tablespoons olive oil

For the tahini sauce:

1 tablespoon maple syrup

Juice of 1 lime

¼ inch fresh ginger, grated

1/3 cup sesame seed paste

Directions:

In a salad bowl, mix the zucchinis with the beets, kale and oil. In another small bowl, whisk the maple syrup with lime juice, ginger and sesame paste. Pour the dressing over the salad, toss and serve it for breakfast.

Enjoy!

Nutrition Values: calories 183, fat 3, fiber 2, carbs 7, protein 9

Quinoa and Spinach Breakfast Salad

Preparation time: 10 minutes

Cooking time: 0 minutes

Servings: 2

Ingredients:

16 ounces quinoa, cooked

1 handful raisins

1 handful baby spinach leaves

1 tablespoon maple syrup

½ tablespoon lemon juice

4 tablespoons olive oil

1 teaspoon ground cumin

A pinch of sea salt and black pepper

½ teaspoon chili flakes

Directions:

In a bowl, mix the quinoa with the spinach, raisins, cumin, salt and pepper and toss. Add the maple syrup, lemon juice, oil and chili flakes and toss then serve for breakfast.

Enjoy!

Nutrition Values: calories 170, fat 3, fiber 6, carbs 8, protein 5

Carrots Breakfast Mix

Preparation time: 10 minutes

Cooking time: 0 minutes

Servings: 4

Ingredients:

1½ tablespoon maple syrup

1 teaspoon olive oil

1 tablespoon chopped walnuts

1 onion, chopped

4 cups shredded carrots

1 tablespoon curry powder

¼ teaspoon ground turmeric

Black pepper to the taste

2 tablespoons sesame seed paste

¼ cup lemon juice

½ cup chopped parsley

Directions:

In a salad bowl, mix together the onion with the carrots, turmeric, curry powder, black pepper, lemon juice and parsley. Add the maple syrup, oil, walnuts and sesame seed paste. toss well and serve for breakfast.

Enjoy!

Nutrition Values: calories 150, fat 3, fiber 2, carbs 6, protein 8

Avocado Omelet

Preparation time: 10 minutes

Cooking time: 10 minutes

Servings: 2

Ingredients:

4 eggs, whisked

2 avocados, pitted, peeled and cubed

A pinch of salt and black pepper

Juice of ½ lemon

1 tablespoon chopped parsley

1 tablespoon olive oil

Directions:

In a bowl, mix the eggs with the avocados, salt, pepper, lemon juice and parsley. Heat up a pan with the oil over medium-high heat then add the avocado and egg mix, spread into the pan and cook for 4 minutes on each side. Divide between plates and serve for breakfast.

Enjoy!

Nutrition Values: calories 201, fat 2, fiber 5, carbs 11, protein 5

Italian Breakfast Salad

Preparation time: 10 minutes

Cooking time: 0 minutes

Servings: 4

Ingredients:

1 handful kalamata olives, pitted and sliced

1 cup cherry tomatoes, halved

1½ cucumbers, sliced

1 red onion, chopped

2 tablespoons chopped oregano

1 tablespoon chopped mint

For the salad dressing:

2 tablespoons balsamic vinegar

¼ cup olive oil

1 garlic clove, minced

2 teaspoons dried Italian herbs

A pinch of salt and black pepper

Directions:

In a salad bowl, toss together the olives with the tomatoes, cucumbers, onion, mint and oregano. In a smaller bowl, whisk the vinegar with the oil, garlic, Italian herbs, salt and pepper. Pour the dressing over the salad, toss and serve for breakfast.

Enjoy!

Nutrition Values: calories 191, fat 10, fiber 3, carbs 13, protein 1

Broccoli and Squash Mix

Preparation time: 10 minutes

Cooking time: 15 minutes

Servings: 4

Ingredients:

4 cups spaghetti squash, peeled, cooked and flesh scrapped out

1½ cups broccoli florets

1 tablespoon olive oil

1 cup coconut milk, unsweetened

1 egg, whisked

1 teaspoon garlic powder

A pinch of salt and black pepper

Directions:

Heat up a pan with the oil over medium-high heat, add the spaghetti squash and the broccoli. Stir and cook for 5-6 minutes. Add the garlic powder, salt, pepper, garlic powder and the egg. Stir and cook for 5 minutes more. Add the coconut milk, mix and cook for about 5 minutes more then divide into bowls and serve for breakfast.

Enjoy!

Nutrition Values: calories 207, fat 5, fiber 8, carbs 14, protein 7

Greens and Berries Mix

Preparation time: 10 minutes

Cooking time: 0 minutes

Servings: 2

Ingredients:

½ cup spinach, torn

½ cup kale, torn

1 cup strawberries, halved

1 cup blueberries

1 banana, peeled and chopped

6 mint leaves, chopped

Directions:

In a bowl, mix the spinach with the kale, strawberries, blueberries, banana and mint. Serve for breakfast.

Enjoy!

Nutrition Values: calories 198, fat 4, fiber 2, carbs 8, protein 6

Veggie and Eggs

Preparation time: 10 minutes

Cooking time: 15 minutes

Servings: 6

Ingredients:

1 red bell pepper, chopped

4 cherry tomatoes, chopped

3 spring onions, chopped

A handful kale, torn

1 tablespoon olive oil

6 eggs

A pinch of salt and black pepper

A pinch of curry powder

Directions:

Heat up a pan with the oil over medium-high heat, add the onions, stir and cook for 1-2 minutes. Add the bell pepper, the tomatoes, the kale, salt, pepper and the curry powder, stir and cook for 4-5 minutes. Crack the eggs into the pan and mix well. Cook until the eggs are done, divide between plates and serve for breakfast.

Enjoy!

Nutrition Values: calories 106, fat 8, fiber 1, carbs 4, protein 7

Coconut Pear Bowl

Preparation time: 10 minutes

Cooking time: 15 minutes

Servings: 4

Ingredients:

2   cups coconut milk, unsweetened

1/3 cup coconut flakes, unsweetened

½ teaspoon vanilla extract

3   pears, peeled, cored and cubed

1.   Directions:

Put the milk in a small pot, add the coconut, vanilla and pears. Stir and bring to a simmer over medium heat, cook for 15 minutes, divide into bowls and serve.

Enjoy!

Nutrition Values: calories 172, fat 5, fiber 7, carbs 8, protein 4

Breakfast Corn Salad

Preparation time: 10 minutes

Cooking time: 0 minutes

Servings: 4

Ingredients:

2 avocados, pitted, peeled and cubed

1-pint mixed cherry tomatoes, halved

2 cups fresh corn kernels

1 red onion, chopped

For the salad dressing:

2 tablespoons olive oil

1 tablespoon lime juice

½ teaspoon grated lime zest

A pinch of salt and black pepper

¼ cup chopped cilantro

Directions:

In a salad bowl, mix the avocados with the tomatoes, corn and onion. Add the oil, lime juice, lime zest, salt, pepper and the cilantro, toss and serve for breakfast.

Nutrition Values: calories 140, fat 3, fiber 2, carbs 6, protein 9

Simple Basil Tomato Mix

Preparation time: 10 minutes

Cooking time: 0 minutes

Servings: 6

Ingredients:

½ cup extra-virgin olive oil

1 cucumber, chopped

2 pints colored cherry tomatoes, halved

Salt and black pepper to the taste

1 red onion, chopped

3 tablespoons red vinegar

1 garlic clove, minced

1 bunch basil, roughly chopped

Directions:

In a salad bowl, toss together the cucumber with the tomatoes, onion, salt, pepper, oil, vinegar, basil and garlic. Serve for breakfast.

Enjoy!

Nutrition Values: calories 100, fat 1, fiber 2, carbs 2, protein 6

Cucumber and Avocado Salad

Preparation time: 10 minutes

Cooking time: 0 minutes

Servings: 4

Ingredients:

1 pound cucumbers, chopped

2 avocados, pitted and chopped

1 small red onion, thinly sliced

2 tablespoons olive oil

2 tablespoons lemon juice

¼ cup chopped parsley

A pinch of salt and black pepper

Directions:

In a salad bowl, mix together the cucumbers with the avocados, onion, oil, lemon juice, parsley, salt and pepper. Serve for breakfast.

Enjoy!

Nutrition Values: calories 120, fat 2, fiber 2, carbs 3, protein 4

Watermelon Salad

Preparation time: 10 minutes

Cooking time: 0 minutes

Servings: 2

Ingredients:

½ teaspoon agave nectar

2 tablespoons lemon juice

1 tablespoon extra-virgin olive oil

1 jalapeno, seeded and chopped

12 ounces watermelon, chopped

1 red onion, thinly sliced

½ cup chopped basil leaves

2 cups baby arugula

Directions:

In a bowl, toss together the watermelon with the jalapeno, onion, basil, arugula, oil, agave nectar, lemon juice and oil. Serve for breakfast.

Nutrition Values: calories 128, fat 8, fiber 2, carbs 16, protein 2

Coconut Porridge

Preparation time: 10 minutes

Cooking time: 15 minutes

Servings: 2

Ingredients:

2 cups coconut milk, unsweetened

3 tablespoons almond flour

½ cup coconut flakes, unsweetened

2 tablespoons ground flax meal

1 teaspoon vanilla extract

2 teaspoons ground cinnamon

Directions:

In a small pot, mix the coconut milk with the almond flour, coconut flakes, flax meal, vanilla and cinnamon. Stir and bring to a simmer over medium heat for 15 minutes. Divide into bowls and serve for breakfast.

Enjoy!

Nutrition Values: calories 287, fat 5, fiber 7, carbs 13, protein 5

Blackberry and Strawberry Salad

Preparation time: 5 minutes

Cooking time: 0 minutes

Servings: 1

Ingredients:

¼ cup sliced almonds

¼ cup blackberries

¼ cup strawberries, halved

1 banana, peeled and sliced

A pinch of ground cinnamon

Directions:

In a bowl, mix the blackberries with strawberries, cinnamon, banana and almonds. Serve for breakfast.

Enjoy!

Nutrition Values: calories 90, fat 3, fiber 1, carbs 0, protein 5

Breakfast Kale Frittata

Preparation time: 10 minutes

Cooking time: 30 minutes

Servings: 4

Ingredients:

6 kale stalks, chopped

1 small sweet onion, chopped

1 small broccoli head, florets separated

2 garlic cloves, minced

Salt and black pepper to the taste

4 eggs

1 tablespoon olive oil

Directions:

Heat up a pan with the oil over medium-high heat, add the onion, stir and cook for 4-5 minutes. Add the garlic, broccoli and kale, toss and cook for 5 minutes more. Add the eggs, salt and pepper and mix. Place in the oven and bake at 380 degrees F for 20 minutes. Slice and serve for breakfast.

Enjoy!

Nutrition Values: calories 214, fat 7, fiber 2, carbs 12, protein 8

Cranberry Granola Bars

Preparation time: 2 hours

Cooking time: 0 minutes

Servings: 4

Ingredients:

2 cups walnuts, toasted

1 cup dates, pitted

3 tablespoons water

¾ cup cranberries, dried, no added sugar

2 cups desiccated coconut, unsweetened

Directions:

In your food processor, mix dates with coconut, cranberries, water and walnuts. Pulse really well then spread the mix into a lined baking dish. Press well into the dish and keep in the fridge for 2 hours then cut into bars and serve.

Enjoy!

Nutrition Values: calories 476, fat 40, fiber 9, carbs 33, protein 6

Spinach and Berry Smoothie

Preparation time: 10 minutes

Cooking time: 0 minutes

Servings: 2

Ingredients:

1 cup blackberries

1 avocado, pitted, peeled and chopped

1 banana, peeled and roughly chopped

1 cup baby spinach

1 tablespoon hemp seeds

1 cup water

½ cup almond milk, unsweetened

Directions:

In your blender, mix the berries with the avocado, banana, spinach, hemp seeds, water and almond milk. Pulse well, divide into 2 glasses and serve for breakfast.

Enjoy!

Nutrition Values: calories 160, fat 3, fiber 4, carbs 6, protein 3

Chapter 10: Lunch Recipes

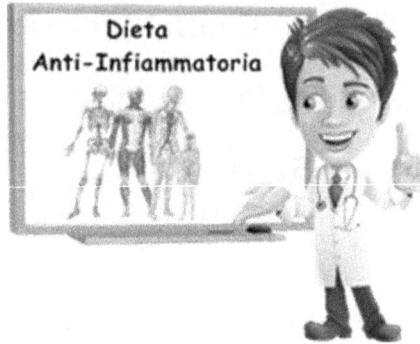

Tasty Grilled Asparagus

Preparation time: 10 minutes

Cooking time: 6 minutes

Servings: 4

Ingredients:

2 pounds asparagus, trimmed

2 tablespoons organic olive oil A

pinch of salt and black pepper

Directions:

In a bowl, combine the asparagus with salt, pepper and oil and toss well.

Place the asparagus on preheated grill over medium-high heat, cook for 3 minutes with them, divide between plates and serve as being a side dish.

Enjoy!

Nutrition Values: calories 172, fat 4, fiber 7, carbs 14, protein 8

Easy Roasted Carrots

Preparation time: ten mins

Cooking time: 30 minutes

Servings: 4

Ingredients:

2 pounds carrots, quartered

A pinch of black pepper

3 tablespoons olive oil

2 tablespoons parsley, chopped

Directions:

Arrange the carrots with a lined baking sheet, add black pepper and oil, toss, introduce inside the oven and cook at 400 degrees F to get a half-hour.

Add parsley, toss, divide between plates and serve as a side dish.

Enjoy!

Nutrition Values: calories 177, fat 3, fiber 6, carbs 14, protein 6

Oven Roasted Asparagus

Preparation time: 10 mins

Cooking time: 25 minutes

Servings: 4

Ingredients:

2 pounds asparagus spears, trimmed

3 tablespoons essential organic olive oil

A pinch of black pepper

2 teaspoons sweet paprika

1 teaspoon sesame seeds

Directions:

Arrange the asparagus on the lined baking sheet, add oil, black pepper and paprika, toss, introduce inside oven and bake at 400 degrees F for 25 minutes.

Divide the asparagus between plates, sprinkle sesame seeds ahead and serve as being a side dish.

Enjoy!

Nutrition Values: calories 190, fat 4, fiber 8, carbs 11, protein 5

Squash Side Salad

Preparation time: 10 minutes

Cooking time: a half-hour

Servings: 6

Ingredients:

1 cup orange juice

3 tablespoons coconut sugar

1 and ½ tablespoons mustard

1 tablespoon ginger, grated

1 and ½ pounds butternut squash, peeled and roughly cubed

Cooking spray

A pinch of black pepper

1/3 cup extra virgin olive oil

6 cups salad greens

1 radicchio, sliced

½ cup pistachios, roasted

Directions:

In a bowl, combine the orange juice with all the sugar, mustard, ginger, black pepper and squash, toss well, spread on a lined baking sheet, spray everything with oil, introduce inside oven and bake at 400 degrees F for thirty minutes.

In a salad bowl, combine the squash with salad greens, radicchio, pistachios and oil, toss well, divide between plates and serve like a side dish.

Enjoy!

Nutrition Values: calories 275, fat 3, fiber 4, carbs 16, protein 6

Colored Iceberg Salad

Preparation time: ten mins

Cooking time: 0 minutes

Servings: 4

Ingredients:

1 iceberg lettuce head, leaves torn

6 bacon slices, cooked and halved

2 green onions, sliced

3 carrots, shredded

6 radishes, sliced

¼ cup red vinegar

¼ cup essential olive oil

3 garlic cloves, minced

A pinch of black pepper

Directions:

In a substantial salad bowl, combine the lettuce leaves with the bacon, green onions, carrots, radishes, vinegar, oil, garlic and black pepper, toss, divide between plates and serve being a side dish.

Enjoy!

Nutrition Values: calories 235, fat 4, fiber 4, carbs 10, protein 6

Fennel Side Salad

Preparation time: ten mins

Cooking time: 0 minutes

Servings: 4

Ingredients:

2 fennel bulbs, trimmed and shaved

1 and ¼ cups zucchini, sliced

2/3 cup dill, chopped

¼ cup freshly squeezed fresh lemon juice

¼ cup essential olive oil

6 cups arugula

½ cups walnuts, chopped

1/3 cup low-fat feta cheese, crumbled

Directions:

In a substantial bowl, combine the fennel while using zucchini, dill, fresh freshly squeezed lemon juice, arugula, oil, walnuts and cheese, toss, divide between plates and serve as a side dish.

Enjoy!

Nutrition Values: calories 188, fat 4, fiber 5, carbs 14, protein 6

Corn Mix

Preparation time: ten minutes

Cooking time: 0 minutes

Servings: 4

Ingredients:

½ cup cider vinegar

¼ cup coconut sugar

A pinch of black pepper

4 cups corn

½ cup red onion, chopped

½ cup cucumber, sliced

½ cup red bell pepper, chopped

½ cup cherry tomatoes, halved

3 tablespoons parsley, chopped

1 tablespoon basil, chopped

1 tablespoon jalapeno, chopped

2 cups baby arugula leaves

Directions:

In a big bowl, combine the corn with onion, cucumber, bell pepper, cherry tomatoes, parsley, basil, jalapeno and arugula and toss.

Add vinegar, sugar and black pepper, toss well, divide between plates and serve just like a side dish.

Enjoy!

Nutrition Values: calories 100, fat 2, fiber 3, carbs 14, protein 4

Persimmon Side Salad

Preparation time: ten mins

Cooking time: 0 minutes

Servings: 4

Ingredients:

Seeds from 1 pomegranate

2 persimmons, cored and sliced

5 cups baby arugula

6 tablespoons green onions, chopped

4 navel oranges, peeled and cut into segments

¼ cup apple cider vinegar

1/3 cup essential olive oil

3 tablespoons pine nuts

1 and ½ teaspoons orange zest, grated

2 tablespoons orange juice

1 tablespoon coconut sugar

½ shallot, chopped

A pinch of cinnamon powder

Directions:

In a salad bowl, combine the pomegranate seeds with persimmons, arugula, green onions and oranges and toss.

In another bowl, combine the vinegar with all the oil, pine nuts, orange zest, orange juice, sugar, shallot and cinnamon, whisk well, add to the salad, toss and serve like a side dish.

Enjoy!

Nutrition Values: calories 188, fat 4, fiber 4, carbs 14, protein 4

Roast green beans with cranberries

Preparation Time: 30 minutes

Servings: 4

Ingredients:

Halved green beans- 2 Ib.

Dried cranberries- ¼ cup

Chopped almonds -¼ cup

Olive oil- 3 tbsp.

Salt

Black pepper

Directions:

Arrange the green beans on a baking sheet and sprinkle oil, salt, and pepper on it.

Mix and roast in the oven for 15 minutes at 425°F.

Stir in the almonds and cranberries and cook for 5 minutes.

Serve.

Nutrition Values:

Calories 181, carbs 10, protein 6, fiber 5, fats 3

Roasted cheesy mushrooms

Preparation Time: 25 minutes

Servings: 4

Ingredients:

Sliced cremini mushrooms- 1½ Ib.

Grated zest of 1 lemon

Grated parmesan - ¼ cup

Dried thyme- 2 tsp.

Minced garlic cloves- 3

Lemon juice- ¼ cup

Olive oil- 3 tbsp.

Salt

Black pepper

Directions:

Coat the baking dish with oil and mix mushrooms with zest, juice, Parmesan, thyme, salt, pepper, and garlic.

Bake in the oven for 15 minutes at 375°F.

Serve.

Nutrition Values:

Calories 199, carbs 12, protein 7, fiber 7, fats 2

Herbed Pork

Preparation time: 10 mins

Cooking time: 60 minutes and 10 minutes

Servings: 6

Ingredients:

2 and ½ pounds pork loin boneless, trimmed and cubed

¾ cup low-sodium chicken stock

2 tablespoons extra virgin extra virgin olive oil

½ tablespoon sweet paprika

2 and ¼ teaspoon sage, dried

½ tablespoon garlic powder

¼ teaspoon rosemary, dried

¼ teaspoon marjoram, dried

1 teaspoon basil, dried

1 teaspoon oregano, dried black pepper

Directions:

In a bowl, mix oil with stock, paprika, garlic powder, sage, rosemary, thyme, marjoram, oregano and pepper for the taste and whisk well.

Heat up a pan over medium-high heat, add the pork and brown it for 5 minutes on either sides.

Add the herbed mix, toss well, cook over medium heat for an hour, divide between plates and serve employing a side salad.

Enjoy!

Nutrition Values: calories 310, fat 4, fiber 6, carbs 12, protein 14

Garlic Pork Shoulder

Preparation time: 10 mins

Cooking time: 4 hours and thirty minutes

Servings: 6

Ingredients:

3 tablespoons garlic, minced

3 tablespoons extra virgin essential olive oil

4 pounds pork shoulder

2 teaspoons sweet paprika

Black pepper for the taste

Directions:

In a bowl, mix extra virgin extra virgin olive oil with paprika, black pepper and oil and whisk well.

Brush pork shoulder with this mix, arrange inside a baking dish and introduce inside oven at 425 degrees for twenty or so minutes.

Reduce heat to 325 degrees F and bake for 4 hours.

Slice the meat, divide it between plates and serve having a side salad.

Enjoy!

Nutrition Values: calories 321, fat 6, fiber 4, carbs 12, protein 18

Pork and Creamy Veggie Sauce

Preparation time: 10 mins

Cooking time: one hour and twenty approximately minutes

Servings: 4

Ingredients:

2 pounds pork roast

1 cup low-sodium veggie stock

2 carrots, chopped

1 leek, chopped

1 celery stalk, chopped

1 teaspoon black peppercorns

2 yellow onions, cut into quarters

1 tablespoon chives, chopped

1 tablespoon parsley, chopped

2 cups nonfat yogurt

1 cup coconut cream

1 teaspoon mustard

Black pepper towards the taste

Directions:

Put the roast in a baking dish, add carrots, leek, celery, peppercorns, onions, stock and black pepper, cover, introduce inside oven and bake at 400 degrees F for sixty minutes and 10 minutes

Transfer the roast using a platter and all sorts of the veggies mix with a pan.

Heat this mix over medium heat, add yogurt, cream and mustard, toss, cook for ten mins, drizzle inside the roast and serve.

Enjoy!

Nutrition Values: calories 263, fat 4, fiber 2, carbs 12, protein 22

Ground Pork Pan

Preparation Time: 10 mins

Cooking time: 20 mins

Servings: 4

Ingredients:

Zest of merely one lemon, grated

Juice of a single lemon

2 garlic cloves, minced

1 tablespoon organic olive oil

1 pound pork meat, ground

Black pepper on the taste

1-pint cherry tomatoes, chopped

1 small red onion, chopped

½ cup low-sodium veggie stock,

2 tablespoons low-sodium tomato paste

1 tablespoon basil, chopped

Directions:

Heat up a pan with all the oil over medium heat, add garlic and onion, stir and cook for 5 minutes.

Add pork, black pepper, tomatoes, stock, freshly squeezed freshly squeezed lemon juice, lemon zest and tomato paste, toss and cook for quarter-hour.

Add basil, toss, divide between plates and serve.

Enjoy!

Nutrition Values: calories 286, fat 8, fiber 7, carbs 14, protein 17

Tarragon Pork Steak

Preparation time: 10 minutes

Cooking time: 22 minutes

Servings: 4

Ingredients:

4 medium pork steaks

Black pepper towards the taste

1 tablespoon extra virgin olive oil

8 cherry tomatoes, halved

A handful tarragon, chopped

Directions:

Heat up a pan while using the oil over medium-high heat, add steaks, season with black pepper, cook them for 6 minutes on each side and divide between plates.

Heat the same pan over medium heat, add the tomatoes along with the tarragon, cook for ten minutes, divide next around the pork and serve.

Enjoy!

Nutrition Values: calories 263, fat 4, fiber 6, carbs 12, protein 16

Pork Meatballs

Preparation time: ten minutes

Cooking time: 10 mins

Servings: 4

Ingredients:

1 pound pork, ground

1/3 cup cilantro, chopped

1 cup red onion, chopped

4 garlic cloves, minced

1 tablespoon ginger, grated

1 Thai chili, chopped

2 tablespoons extra virgin olive oil

Directions:

In a bowl, combine the meat with cilantro, onion, garlic, ginger and chili, stir well and shape medium meatballs out of this mix.

Heat up a pan while using oil over medium-high heat, add the meatballs, cook them for 5 minutes on either side, divide them between plates and serve with a side salad.

Enjoy!

Nutrition Values: calories 220, fat 4, fiber 2, carbs 8, protein 14

Nutmeg Meatballs Curry

Preparation Time: 40 minutes

Servings: 3

Ingredients:

Pork meat, ground- 2/3 lbs.

Egg -½

Parsley, chopped-1 tbsp

Coconut flour-2 tbsp

Garlic clove, minced-1

Salt and black pepper - to taste

Veggie stock -¼ cup

Tomato passata-½ cup

Nutmeg, ground -¼ tsp

Sweet paprika -¼ tsp

Olive oil-1 tbsp

Carrot, chopped -1

Directions:

Thoroughly mix the meat with egg, parsley, salt, pepper, garlic, nutmeg, and paprika in a suitable bowl.

Mix well and make small meatballs out of this mixture.

Dredge these balls through dry flour or dust the balls with flour.

Place a pot with oil over medium-high heat.

Add dusted meatballs in the pot and sear them for 4 minutes per side.

Toss in tomato passata, carrots, and stock.

Cover this mixture and let it simmer for 20 minutes.

Serve right away.

Devour.

Nutrition Values:

Calories: 281, Fat: 8, Fiber: 6, Carbs: 10, Protein: 15

Pan seared sausage and kale

Preparation Time: 35 minutes

Servings: 4

Ingredients:

Chopped kale- 5 Ib.

Italian pork sausage: sliced- 1½ Ib.

Minced garlic- 1 tsp.

Water- 1 cup

Onion: chopped- 1 cup

Red bell pepper: seeded and chopped ½ cup

Red chili pepper: chopped ½ cup

Black pepper

Salt

Directions:

Put a pan on medium heat and add the sausage to brown for 10 minutes.

Mix in onions and town for 3-4 minutes.

Add in the garlic and bell pepper and cook for 1 minute.

Mix in the chili, kale, water, pepper and salt and let cook for 10 minutes.

Serve

Nutrition Values:

Calories- 872, carbs- 61, protein- 54, fiber- 3, fats- 43

Pan-Fried Chorizo Mix

Preparation Time: 35 minutes

Servings: 4

Ingredients:

Chopped tomato, 1

Olive oil, 1 tbsp.

Sugar-free chorizo sausages, 2

Chopped zucchini, 1

Chopped red bell pepper, 1

Minced garlic cloves, 2

Black pepper

Chicken stock, 2 cup.

Chopped parsley, 2 tbsps.

Lemon juice, 1 tbsp.

Salt

Chopped yellow onion, 1

Directions:

Set the pan on fire to fry the chorizo and onion for 3 minutes over medium-high heat.

Stir in the bell pepper, garlic, lemon juice, tomato, pepper, stock, and salt.

Allow to simmer for 10 minutes while covered

Mix in the zucchini and parsley to cook for 12 minutes.

Set in serving bowls and enjoy

Nutrition Values:

Calories: 280, Fat: 8, Fiber: 3, Carbs: 5, Protein: 17

Pork Rolls

Preparation Time: 30 minutes

Servings: 6

Ingredients:

3 Peeled and minced garlic cloves

Italian seasoning - ½ teaspoon

6 prosciutto slices

Chopped fresh parsley - 2 tablespoons

Thinly sliced pork cutlets- 1 pound

Coconut oil - 1 tablespoon

Chopped onion- ¼ cup

Canned diced tomatoes - 15 ounces

Chicken stock - ⅓ cup

Grated Parmesan cheese - 2 tablespoons

Ricotta cheese- ⅓ cup e

Seasoning: Salt and ground black pepper

Directions:

Flatten pork pieces with a meat pounder.

Put prosciutto slices on top of each piece and then divide ricotta cheese, parsley, and Parmesan cheese.

Each piece of pork should be rolled and secure with a toothpick.

With medium-high temperature, heat the oil in a pan, add pork rolls, cook until brown on both sides, and transfer to a plate.

Heat the pan again over medium temperature, put onion and garlic, mix well. Cook for 5 minutes.

The stock should be added and cook for another 3 minutes.

Remove toothpicks from pork rolls and return into the pan.

Put tomatoes, Italian seasoning, salt, and pepper, bring to commotion by stirring, bring to a boil, reduce heat to medium-low, cover the pan with lid, and cook for 30 minutes.

Divide between plates and serve it.

Nutrition Values:

Calories: 256, Fat: 19, Fiber: 1, Carbs: 17, Protein: 12

Salad Bowl of CapreseWith Tomato

Preparation Time: 7 minutes

Servings: 3

Ingredients:

Mozzarella cheese-1/2 pound (sliced)

Balsamic vinegar-1 tablespoon

Olive oil-1 tablespoon

Tomato-1 (sliced)

Basil leaves-4 (torn)

Salt and black pepper-To taste

Instructions:

Settle the tomato and mozzarella slices alternatively.

Display on 2 plates. Season with the salt and pepper.

Drizzle the vinegar and olive oil. Sprinkle the basil leaves at the end.

Serve.

Nutrition :

Calories:- 150; Fat : 12; Fiber : 5; Carbs : 6; Protein : 9

Sauté Cabbage with Butter

Preparation and Cooking Time 20 minutes.

Servings: 4

Ingredients:

Green cabbage, shredded: 1½ pound

Salt: to taste

Ground black pepper: to taste

Unsalted butter: 5 ounces

Sweet paprika: 1/8 teaspoon

Directions:

Place a medium skillet pan over medium heat, add butter and when it melts, add cabbage.

Cook cabbage for 15 minutes, stirring often and then season with salt, black pepper, and paprika.

Continue cooking for 1 minute, then divide evenly between plates and serve.

Nutrition Values:

Calories: 805, Fat: 84, Fiber: 3, Carbs: 9, Protein: 1

Saute Edamame with Mint

Preparation and Cooking Time 10 minutes

Servings: 4

Ingredients:

Edamame: ¾ pound

Salt: to taste

Ground black pepper: to taste

Mint leaves, chopped: 1 tablespoon

Olive oil: 2 teaspoons

Green onions, chopped: 3

Minced garlic: ½ teaspoon

Directions:

Place a pan over medium heat, add oil and when hot, add edamame beans.

Season with salt and black pepper, then add remaining ingredients and stir until well mixed.

Cook edamame for 5 minutes until heated through, then divide evenly between serving plates and serve.

Nutrition Values:

Calories: 91, Fat: 3, Fiber: 4, Carbs: 17, Protein: 7

Sauteed Broccoli with Parmesan

Preparation Time: 32 minutes

Servings: 4

Ingredients:

broccoli florets - 1 pound

garlic clove - 1, minced

parmesan - 1 tablespoon, grated

olive oil - 5 tablespoons

Salt and black pepper to the taste.

Instructions:

Pour some water in a pot, then add a little salt and bring to a boil over medium high heat source.

Then add broccoli, cook for 5 minutes before removing the water.

Heat up a pan containing the oil over medium high heat source; then add garlic. Stir and cook for about 2 more minutes

Add broccoli; stir and cook for another 15 minutes

Remove the heat; sprinkle parmesan.

Divide into clean plates and serve

Nutrition :

Calories:- 193; Fat : 14; Fiber : 3; Carbs : 6; Protein : 5

Sautéed Kohlrabi with Parsley

Preparation and Cooking Time 15 minutes

Servings: 4

Ingredients:

Kohlrabi, trimmed and sliced thin: 2

Salt: to taste

Ground black pepper: to taste

Chopped parsley: 1 tablespoon

Unsalted butter: 1 tablespoon

Minced garlic: 1 teaspoon

Directions:

Place kohlrabi in a medium saucepan, pour in enough water to cover it, then place the pan over medium heat and bring to boil.

Then cook for 5 minutes, drain kohlrabi and transfer into a bowl.

Place a medium skillet pan over medium heat, add butter and when it melts, add garlic and cook for 1 minute or until fragrant.

Add kohlrabi, season with salt and black pepper and cook for 3 minutes per side or until nicely golden brown on both sides.

Add parsley, toss until mixed and remove pan from heat.

Divide kohlrabi evenly between serving plates and serve straight away.

Nutrition Values:

Calories: 55, Fat: 3, Fiber: 7, Carbs: 8, Protein: 9

Sautéed Mixed Vegetable with Pumpkin Seeds

Preparation and Cooking Time 10 minutes

Servings: 4

Ingredients:

Mushrooms, sliced: 14 ounces

Broccoli florets: 3 ounces

Red bell pepper, seeded and cut into strips: 3 ounces

Spinach, torn: 3 ounces

Garlic, minced: 2 tablespoons

Salt: to taste

Ground black pepper: to taste

Red pepper flakes: 1/8 teaspoon

Olive oil: 6 tablespoons

Pumpkin seeds: 2 tablespoons

Directions:

Place a skillet pan over medium-high heat, add oil and when hot, add garlic and cook for 1 minute or until fragrant.

Add mushrooms and cook for 3 minutes.

Then add broccoli florets and pepper, stir well, season with salt and black pepper, add pepper flakes and pumpkin seeds and cook for 3 minutes.

Add spinach, stir until just mixed, cook for 3 minutes and remove the pan from heat.

Serve straightaway.

Nutrition Values:

Calories: 271, Fat: 27, Fiber: 5, Carbs: 14, Protein: 6

Side Cauliflower Salad

Preparation Time: 15 minutes

Servings: 10

Ingredients:

Mayonnaise. 1 c

Salt

Chopped hard-boiled eggs, 4

Black pepper

Chopped celery, 1 cup.

Cauliflower florets, 21 oz.

Cider vinegar, 2 tbsps.

Erythritol, 1 tsp.

Water, 1 tbsp.

Chopped onion, 1 cup.

Directions:

Microwave the cauliflower florets with water in a heatproof bowl for 5 minutes

Set the salad in a bowl

Mix in the onions, celery, and eggs as you stir gently.

Combine salt, mayonnaise, pepper, vinegar, and erythritol in another bowl.

Add the mixture to the cauliflower, toss and enjoy.

Nutrition Values:

Calories: 139, Fat: 7, Fiber: 9, Carbs: 18, Protein: 8

Spicy Green Beans and Vinaigrette

Preparation Time: 22 minutes

Servings: 8

Ingredients:

Minced garlic clove, 1

Macadamia nut oil, 4 tbsps.

Lemon juice, 1 tsp.

Green beans, 2 lbs.

Smoked paprika, 2 tsps.

Salt

Chopped chorizo, 2 oz.

Black pepper

Coconut oil, 2 tbsps.

Coriander, ¼ tsp.

Beef stock, 2 tbsps.

Coconut vinegar, ½ cup.

Directions:

Put lemon juice, chorizo, vinegar, pepper, paprika, garlic, and salt in a blender to pulse until smooth.

Mix in macadamia nut oil and stock to blend again

Allow the coconut oil to melt over medium heat to sauté the green beans and chorizo mixture.

Cook for 10 minutes as you stir gently

Enjoy this wonderful meal

Nutrition Values:

Calories: 159, Fat: 11, Fiber: 1, Carbs: 8, Protein: 9

Stuffed Sausage with Bacon Wrappings

Preparation Time: 40 minutes

Servings: 4

Ingredients:

Onion powder

Bacon strips,

Salt.

Garlic powder.

Black pepper.

Sausages,

Sweet paprika, ½ tsp.

Pepper jack cheese slices, 1

Directions:

Ensure you have a medium high source of heat. Set a grill on it. Add sausages to cook until done all sides and set on a plate to cool.

Slice a pocket opening in the sausages. Each to be stuffed with 2 slices of pepper jack cheese. Apply a seasoning of onion, pepper, garlic powder, paprika and salt.

Each stuffed sausage should be wrapped in a bacon strip and grip using a toothpick. Set them on the baking sheet and transfer to the oven to bake at 400 0F for almost 15 minutes.

Serve immediately and enjoy.

Nutrition :

calories: 500, fat: 37, fiber: 12, carbs: 4, protein: 40

Tasty Lunch Pizza

Preparation Time: 17 minutes

Servings: 4

Ingredients:

Mascarpone cheese, ¼ cup.

Clive oil, 1 tbsp.

Shredded pizza cheese mix, 1 cup.

Ghee, 2 tbsps.

Heavy cream, 1 tbsp.

Lemon pepper

Shredded mozzarella cheese, 1 cup.

Steamed broccoli florets, 1/3 cup.

Salt.

Minced garlic, 1 tsp.

Black pepper.

Shaved asiago cheese

Directions:

Set the pan on fire to heat the oil to cook pizza mix then spread into a circle over medium heat

Spread the mozzarella cheese into a circle also

Allow everything to cook for 5 minutes and set on a plate

Set the pan on fire to melt the ghee for cooking lemon pepper, mascarpone cheese, cream, salt, pepper, and garlic for 5 minutes over medium heat.

Spread half of this mix over cheese crust.

Mix in broccoli florets to the pan with the remaining mascarpone mix to cook for 1 minute

Top the mixture on the pizza, sprinkle asiago cheese at the end and serve

Nutritional :

calories: 250, fat: 15, fiber: 1, carbs: 3, protein: 10

Turkey and Collard Greens Soup

Preparation and Cooking Time 2 hours and 30 minutes

Servings: 10

Ingredients:

Collard greens, chopped: 5 bunches

Salt: to taste

Ground black pepper: to taste

Red pepper flakes: 1 tablespoon

Chicken stock: 5 cups

Turkey leg: 1

Minced garlic: 2 tablespoons

Olive oil: ¼ cup

Directions:

Place a large pot over medium heat, add oil and when hot, add garlic.

Cook garlic for 1 minute, then turkey, season with salt and black pepper and then pout in stock.

Stir the mixture and simmer the soup for 30 minutes, covering the pot.

Add collard greens, stir until just mixed and cook for 45 minutes, covering the pot.

Then reduce heat to medium level, taste soup to adjust seasoning and continue cooking for 1 hour, covering the pot.

When done, take out greens from the soup using a slotted spoon, then take out the chicken and transfer to a cutting board.

Let the turkey cool for 10 minutes, then chop into bite size pieces and add into the soup.

Return greens into the soup, season with red pepper flakes and ladle evenly into serving bowls.

Serve immediately.

Nutrition Values:

Calories: 171, Fat: 19, Fiber: 8, Carbs: 2, Protein: 11

Warm Delicious Roasted Olives

Preparation Time: 30 minutes

Servings: 6

Ingredients:

kalamata olives - 1 cup, pitted

black olives - 1 cup, pitted

garlic cloves - 10

herbs de Provence - 1 tablespoon

lemon zest - 1 teaspoon, grated

green olives - 1 cup, stuffed with almonds and garlic

olive oil - 1/4 cup

Black pepper to the taste.

Some chopped thyme for serving

Instructions:

Spread black, kalamata and green olives on a lined baking sheet neatly, and drizzle some oil on them as well as on garlic and herbs de Provence,

Then toss to keep it well coated. Transfer into an oven set at a temperature of 425 0F and bake for 10 minutes

Stir the olives and bake for 10 another minutes.

Cut the olives on different plates, sprinkle lemon zest, black pepper and thyme on top.

Toss to ensure it is coated. Serve warm.

Nutrition :

Calories:- 200; Fat : 20; Fiber : 4; Carbs : 3; Protein : 1

Yummy Creamy Spaghetti Pasta: Side Dish

Preparation Time: 50 minutes

Servings: 4

Ingredients:

spaghetti squash - 1

ghee - 2 tablespoons

heavy cream - 2 cups

Cajun seasoning - 1 teaspoon

A pinch of cayenne pepper

Salt and black pepper to the taste.

Instructions:

Prick spaghetti with a fork, then arrange neatly on a lined baking sheet.

Move to an oven at 350 0F and bake for 15 minutes

Remove the spaghetti squash from the oven, keep it aside for a while and let it cool down. Scoop squash noodles

Heat up a pan containing ghee over medium heat; before adding spaghetti squash.

Then stir gently and cook for a couple of minutes

Sprinkle a pinch of salt, pepper, cayenne pepper and Cajun seasoning.

Then stir and cook for about a minute

Add heavy cream; stir, cook for 10 another 10 minutes.

Cut into different plates and serve as a keto side dish.

Nutrition :

Calories:- 200; Fat : 2; Fiber : 1; Carbs : 5; Protein : 8

Yummy Muffins

Preparation Time: 55 minutes

Servings: 13

Ingredients:

Egg yolks, 6

Coconut flour, ¾ cup.

Mushrooms, ½ lb.

Salt.

Ground beef, 1 lb.

Coconut aminos, 2 tbsps.

Directions:

Combine egg yolks, coconut aminos and salt in a blender. Process well until the desired consistency is attained.

In a separate bowl, stir in salt and beef. Stir in mushroom mixture to combine.

Stir in coconut flour.

Set the mixture into 13 cupcake cups and transfer into an oven preheated at 350 0F. bake the cups until done for 45 minutes

Allow to cool and enjoy your lunch

Nutritional :

calories: 160, fiber: 3, carbs: 1, fat: 10, protein: 12

Zucchini and Squash Noodles with Peppers

Preparation and Cooking Time 30 minutes

Servings: 6

Ingredients:

Medium zucchinis, cut with a spiralizer: 1 ½

Medium summer squash, cut with a spiralizer: 1

Butternut squash, cut with a spiralizer: 4 ounce

Medium white onion, peeled and chopped: 4 ounces

Mixed bell peppers, seeded and cut into thin strips: 6 ounces

Minced garlic: 1 ½ teaspoon

Salt: to taste

Ground black pepper: to taste

Bacon fat: 4 tablespoons

Directions:

Set oven to 400 0F and let preheat.

In the meantime, place zucchini noodles on a baking sheet lined with parchment paper and then add onion and bell peppers.

Add garlic, season with salt and black pepper and toss until evenly coated.

Add bacon fat, toss until coated and place the baking sheet into an oven.

Bake for 20 minutes or until done and serve straightaway.

Nutrition Values:

Calories: 179, Fat: 6, Fiber: 6, Carbs: 19, Protein: 10

Baked Potato Mix

Preparation time: 10 mins

Cooking time: one hour and quarter-hour

Servings: 8

Ingredients:

6 potatoes, peeled and sliced

2 garlic cloves, minced

2 tablespoons organic olive oil

1 and ½ cups coconut cream

¼ cup coconut milk

1 tablespoon thyme, chopped

¼ teaspoon nutmeg, ground

A pinch of red pepper flakes

1 and ½ cups low-fat cheddar, shredded

½ cup low-fat parmesan, grated

Directions:

Heat up a pan with all the oil over medium heat, add garlic, stir and cook for 1 minute.

Add coconut cream, coconut milk, thyme, nutmeg and pepper flakes, stir, bring which has a simmer, reduce heat to low and cook for 10 mins.

Arrange 1/3 with all the potatoes in a very baking dish, add 1/3 with the cream, repeat with the rest through the potatoes along with the cream, sprinkle the cheddar for the top, cover with tin foil, introduce within the oven and cook at 375 degrees F for 45 minutes.

Uncover the dish, sprinkle the parmesan, bake everything for 20 mins, divide between plates and serve as as being a side dish.

Enjoy!

Nutrition Values: calories 224, fat 8, fiber 9, carbs 16, protein 15

Spicy Brussels sprouts

Preparation time: ten mins

Cooking time: 20 minutes

Servings: 6

Ingredients:

2 pounds Brussels sprouts, halved

2 tablespoons essential extra virgin olive oil

A pinch of black pepper

1 tablespoon sesame oil

2 garlic cloves, minced

½ cup coconut aminos

2 teaspoons apple cider vinegar treatment

1 tablespoon coconut sugar

2 teaspoons chili sauce

A pinch of red pepper flakes

Sesame seeds for serving

Directions:

Spread the sprouts over the lined baking dish, add the primary essential olive oil, the sesame oil, black pepper, garlic, aminos, vinegar, coconut sugar, chili sauce and pepper flakes, toss well, introduce within the oven and bake at 425 degrees F for twenty minutes.

Divide the sprouts between plates, sprinkle sesame seeds at the very top and serve as a side dish.

Enjoy!

Nutrition Values: calories 176, fat 3, fiber 6, carbs 14, protein 9

Baked Cauliflower

Preparation time: ten minutes

Cooking time: half an hour

Servings: 4

Ingredients:

3 tablespoons organic extra virgin olive oil

2 tablespoons chili sauce

Juice of a single lime

3 garlic cloves, minced

1 cauliflower head, florets separated

A pinch of black pepper

1 teaspoon cilantro, chopped

Directions:

In a bowl, combine the oil while using chili sauce, lime juice, garlic and black pepper and whisk.

Add cauliflower florets, toss, spread on the lined baking sheet, introduce inside oven and bake at 425 degrees F for a half-hour.

Divide the cauliflower between plates, sprinkle cilantro at the top and serve as being a side dish.

Enjoy!

Nutrition Values: calories 188, fat 4, fiber 7, carbs 14, protein 8

Baked Broccoli

Preparation time: ten minutes

Cooking time: quarter-hour

Servings: 4

Ingredients:

1 tablespoon organic olive oil

1 broccoli head, florets separated

2 garlic cloves, minced

½ cup coconut cream

½ cup low-fat mozzarella, shredded

¼ cup low-fat parmesan, grated

A pinch of pepper flakes, crushed

Directions:

In a baking dish, combine the broccoli with oil, garlic, cream, pepper flakes and mozzarella and toss.

Sprinkle the parmesan on top, introduce inside the oven and bake at 375 degrees F for fifteen minutes.

Divide between plates and serve as a side dish.

Enjoy!

Nutrition Values: calories 188, fat 4, fiber 7, carbs 14, protein 7

Easy Slow Cooked Potatoes

Preparation time: 10 mins

Cooking time: 6 hours

Servings: 6

Ingredients:

Cooking spray

2   pounds baby potatoes, quartered

3 cups low-fat cheddar cheese, shredded

2 garlic cloves, minced

8 bacon slices, cooked and chopped

¼ cup green onions, chopped

1 tablespoon sweet paprika

A pinch of black pepper

Directions:

Spray a pokey cooker while using cooking spray, add baby potatoes, cheddar, garlic, bacon, green onions, paprika and black pepper, toss, cover and cook on High for 6 hours.

Divide between plates and serve being a side dish.

Enjoy!

Nutrition Values: calories 200, fat 4, fiber 6, carbs 12, protein 7

Mashed Potatoes

Preparation time: 10 minutes

Cooking time: 20 mins

Servings: 6

Ingredients:

3 pounds potatoes, peeled and cubed

2 tablespoons non-fat butter

½ cup coconut milk

A pinch of salt and black pepper

½ cup low-fat sour cream

Directions:

Put the potatoes in the pot, add water to purchase, put in a pinch of salt and pepper, bring with a boil over medium heat, cook for twenty or so minutes and drain.

Add butter, milk and sour cream, mash well, stir everything, divide between plates and serve as a side dish.

Enjoy!

Nutrition Values: calories 188, fat 3, fiber 7, carbs 14, protein 8

Avocado Side Salad

Preparation time: ten mins

Cooking time: 0 minutes

Servings: 4

Ingredients:

4 blood oranges, peeled and cut into segments

2 tablespoons extra virgin olive oil

A pinch of red pepper, crushed

2 avocados, peeled, pitted and cut into wedges

1 and ½ cups baby arugula

¼ cup almonds, toasted and chopped

1 tablespoon fresh freshly squeezed lemon juice

Directions:

In a bowl, combine the oranges while using oil, red pepper, avocados, arugula, almonds and fresh lemon juice, toss, divide between plates and serve as being a side dish.

Enjoy!

Nutrition Values: calories 231, fat 4, fiber 8, carbs 16, protein 6

Classic Side Dish Salad

Preparation time: ten mins

Cooking time: 0 minutes

Servings: 4

Ingredients:

3 garlic cloves, minced

Juice of ½ lemon

6 ounces coconut cream

2 lettuce hearts, torn

1 cup corn

4 ounces green beans, halved

1 cup cherry tomatoes, halved

1 cucumber, chopped

1/3 cup chives, chopped

1 avocado, peeled, pitted and halved

6 bacon slices, cooked and chopped

Directions:

In a bowl, combine the lettuce with corn, green beans, cherry tomatoes, cucumber, chives, avocado and bacon and toss.

In another bowl, combine the garlic with fresh fresh lemon juice and coconut cream, whisk well, add towards the salad, toss and serve as a side dish.

Enjoy!

Nutrition Values: calories 175, fat 12, fiber 4, carbs 13, protein 6

Easy Kale Mix

Preparation time: ten mins

Cooking time: 0 minutes

Servings: 4

Ingredients:

1 wheat grains bread slice, toasted and torn into small pieces

6 tablespoons low-fat cheddar, grated

3 tablespoons extra virgin olive oil

5 tablespoons fresh lemon juice

1 garlic herb, minced

7 cups kale, torn

A pinch of black pepper

Directions:

In a bowl, combine the bread with cheese and kale.

In another bowl, combine the oil with all the freshly squeezed lemon juice, garlic and black pepper, whisk, add towards the salad, toss, divide between plates and serve as as a side dish.

Enjoy!

Nutrition Values: calories 200, fat 4, fiber 5, carbs 14, protein 8

Asparagus Salad

Preparation time: ten mins

Cooking time: 4 minutes

Servings: 4

Ingredients:

4 tablespoons avocado oil

2 tablespoons balsamic vinegar

1 tablespoon coconut aminos

1 garlic herb, minced

1 pound asparagus, trimmed

6 cups frisee lettuce leaves, torn

1 cup edamame, shelled

1 cup parsley, chopped

Directions:

Heat up a pan with 1 tablespoon oil over medium-high heat, add asparagus, cook for 4 minutes and transfer which has a salad bowl.

Add lettuce, edammae and parsley and toss.

In another bowl, combine the remaining from your oil when using vinegar, aminos and garlic, whisk well, add inside the salad, toss, divide between plates and serve as being a side dish.

Enjoy!

Nutrition Values: calories 200, fat 4, fiber 5, carbs 14, protein 6

Green Side Salad

Preparation time: 10 minutes

Cooking time: 0 minutes

Servings: 4

Ingredients:

4 cups baby spinach leaves

1 cucumber, sliced

3 ounces broccoli florets

3 ounces green beans, blanched and halved

¾ cup edamame, shelled

1 and ½ cups green grapes, halved

1 cup orange juice

¼ cup extra virgin organic olive oil

1 tablespoon cider vinegar

2 tablespoons parsley, chopped

2 teaspoons mustard

A pinch of black pepper

Directions:

In a salad bowl, combine a baby spinach with cucumber, broccoli, green beans, edamame and grapes and toss.

Add orange juice, organic extra virgin olive oil, vinegar, parsley, mustard and black pepper, toss well, divide between plates and serve as a side dish.

Enjoy!

Nutrition Values: calories 117, fat 4, fiber 5, carbs 14, protein 4

Baked Zucchini

Preparation time: ten mins

Cooking time: 20 minutes

Servings: 4

Ingredients:

4 zucchinis, quartered lengthwise

½ teaspoon thyme, dried

½ teaspoon oregano, dried

½ cup low-fat parmesan, grated

½ teaspoon basil, dried

¼ teaspoon garlic powder

2 tablespoons essential olive oil

2 tablespoons parsley, chopped

A pinch of black pepper

Directions:

Arrange zucchini pieces having a lined baking sheet, add thyme, oregano, basil, garlic powder, oil, parsley and black pepper and toss well.

Sprinkle parmesan ahead, introduce within the oven and bake at 350 degrees F for twenty roughly minutes.

Divide between plates and serve as a side dish.

Enjoy!

Nutrition Values: calories 198, fat 4, fiber 4, carbs 14, protein 5

Chapter 11 : Dinner Recipes

Biryani

Servings: 6

Preparation Time: 15 minutes

Cooking Time: 15 minutes

Total Time: 30 minutes

Ingredients

Black pepper as desired

Sea salt as desired

Garam masala .5 tsp

Coconut oil 1 tsp

Shelled peas 1 c

Water 5 c

Coriander .5 tsp ground

Chili powder 1 tsp

Turmeric 5 tsp

Carrots 2 quartered

Potatoes 2 quartered

Bay leaves 2 torn

Cumin seeds .5 tsp

Onion 1 sliced thin

Vegetable oil 3 T

White rice long grain 2 c

Directions

Add the rice to a large pot and cover it with three to four inches of water before allowing it to soak for about 20 minutes. Drain and set aside.

Add the oil to your pressure cooker and set it over medium heat. Add in the onion, bay leaves, and cumin seeds and let everything cook about 5 minutes until the onion is nearly see through.

Mix in the carrots and potatoes and let them cook an additional 5 minutes and the potatoes have begun to brown. Add in the coriander, turmeric and chili powder and let everything cook 1 additional minute.

Add the rice to the pressure cooker and ensure it is well covered in the boil before adding in the peas and water. Mix in the garam masala, oil, and salt before sealing the cooker and turning it to high pressure. Let everything cook for 5 minutes before removing from heat.

Allow the pressure to naturally release and fluff the rice with a fork prior to serving.

Autumn Roasted Green Beans

Servings: 4

Preparation Time: 15 minutes

Cooking Time: 30 minutes

Total Time: 45 minutes

Ingredients

Walnuts .5 c toasted

Cranberries .5 c dried

Black pepper as desired

Kosher sea salt as desired

Lemon juice 2 tsp.

Lemon zest 1 tsp.

Sugar .25 tsp.

Coconut oil 2 T

Garlic 4 cloves, quartered and peeled

Green beans 2 lbs. stems trimmed

Directions

Preheat your oven to 350F and crack and smash the walnuts into chunks.

Spread the walnuts onto a baking sheet and toast them for 10 minutes.

Increase the temperature on the oven to 450F.

Cover a baking sheet with a rim using aluminum foil.

In a mixing bowl, combine the sugar, pepper, salt and coconut oil before coating the garlic and green beans thoroughly.

Place the beans onto a baking sheet and spread them out to ensure they cook well. Place the sheet into the oven and let the beans bake for 15 minutes, before stirring with a spatula and roasting another 10 minutes.

Mix in the lemon juice, pepper and salt prior to serving.

Zoodles

Servings: 2

Preparation Time: 5 minutes

Cooking Time: 0 minutes

Total Time: 5 minutes

Ingredients

Zucchini 4 organic

Directions- Zoodle Creation

If you have access to a spiralizer, use it to create noodles of zucchini. If you do not own a spiralizer, this recipe is still very simple. Just slice the zucchini into long thin strips. You may also wish to use a cheese and vegetable grater to get the desired noodle effect.

Serve the zoodles as they are or let them boil for two minutes in a pan of water to warm them up and soften them a bit. Alternately, you may wish to sauté them in a bit of coconut oil or Coconut oil for a minute or two to give them a little crispness.

Serve the zoodles in place of the traditional noodles in your favorite pasta dishes.

Roasted Rosemary Potatoes

Servings: 6

Preparation Time: 10 minutes

Cooking Time: 25 minutes

Total Time: 35 minutes

Ingredients

Garlic 1 head

Rosemary 3 sprigs

Thyme 3 sprigs

Baby potatoes 20 oz.

Parsley 2 T chopped

Sea salt as desired

Black pepper as desired

Coconut oil 2 T

Directions

Ensure your oven is heated to 450F.

Separate garlic cloves and remove the papery skin holding them together, but do not peel.

Add the rosemary, thyme, baby potatoes, parsley, garlic, and coconut oil together in a large bowl, coating well.

Add the results to a jelly roll pan that has been lined with tinfoil before topping with pepper and salt. Place the pan in the oven and let the potatoes bake approximately 25 minutes, stirring at the 12-minute mark.

Season with additional pepper and salt prior to serving.

Sweet Potato Wedges

Servings: 6

Preparation Time: 10 minutes

Cooking Time: 30 minutes

Total Time: 40 minutes

Ingredients

Salt 1 tsp.

Cracked black pepper 1 tsp.

Garlic powder .5 tsp.

Sweet potatoes 4 medium, peeled, each cut into 6 wedges

Rosemary 1 T chopped, fresh

Coconut oil 2 T

Directions

Preheat oven to 450F.

In a mixing bowl, combine the coconut oil, rosemary, sweet potatoes, garlic powder, black pepper, and salt together and ensure the potatoes are coated well.

Add the results in a single layer to a large roasting pan before placing the pan in the oven and letting the potatoes bake for 20 minutes. Turn the dish at this point before baking another 10 minutes.

Best Lentil Curry

Servings: 4

Preparation Time: 10 min

Cooking Time: 30 minutes

Total Time: 40 minutes

Ingredients

Vegetable broth 4 c low sodium

Red lentil 1 c

Potato 10 oz. peeled and made into pieces that are 1 inch each

Carrot 8 oz. chopped

Curry powder 1 T

Scallions 8 separated, sliced

Garlic 2 cloves chopped

Ginger 2 T chopped

Coconut oil 3 T

Directions

- Add the oil to a saucepan before placing it on the stove on top of a burner set to a high/medium heat.

- Add in the scallion whites, garlic and ginger and let them soften for 2 minutes.

- Mix in the curry powder as well as pepper and salt, as desired, broth, lentils, potato, and carrots before letting everything boil. Turn down the heat and let everything simmer for 15 minutes, stirring regularly.

- Top with scallion greens prior to serving.

Parmesan sprinkled garlic beans

Preparation Time: 20 minutes

Servings: 4

Ingredients:

Trimmed green beans- 1½ Ib.

Olive oil- 3 tbsp.

Minced garlic cloves- 4

Grated parmesan: 2 tbsp.

Red pepper flakes- ½ tsp.

Directions:

Cover beans with water in a pot and simmer over medium-high for 5 minutes.

Remove the water and set aside in a bowl.

Pour oil in a an over medium-high and add pepper flakes, garlic, and beans an cook for 6 minutes.

Serve topped with parmesan.

Nutrition Values:

Calories 200, carbs 11, protein 6, fiber 6, fats 3

Lamb & Pineapple Kebabs

One of the delicious recipe of lamb and pineapple kebabs with a tasty layer of char... Fresh mint gives a refreshing touch to these kebabs.

Servings: 4-6

Preparation Time: 15 minutes

Cooking Time: 10 minutes

Ingredients:

1 large pineapple, cubed into 1½-inch size, divided

1 (½-inch) piece fresh ginger, chopped

2 garlic cloves, chopped

Salt, to taste

16-24-ounce lamb shoulder steak, trimmed and cubed into 1½-inch size

Fresh mint leaves from a bunch

Ground cinnamon, to taste

Directions:

In a food processor, add about 1½ cups of pineapple, ginger, garlic and salt and pulse till smooth.

Transfer the mixture into a large bowl.

Add chops and coat with mixture generously.

Refrigerate to marinate for about 1-2 hours.

Preheat the grill to medium heat. Grease the grill grate.

Thread lam, remaining pineapple and mint leaves onto pre-soaked wooden skewers.

Grill the kebabs for about 10 minutes, turning occasionally.

Baked Meatballs & Scallions

A recipe of lamb meatballs that is filled with flavor and aroma... Baked meatballs pair nicely with the crispy tips of braised scallions.

Servings: 4-6

Preparation Time: 20 minutes

Cooking Time: 35 minutes

Ingredients:

For Meatballs:

1 lemongrass stalk, outer skin peeled and chopped

1 (1½-inch) piece fresh ginger, sliced

3 garlic cloves, chopped

1 cup fresh cilantro leaves, chopped roughly

½ cup fresh basil leaves, chopped roughly

2 tablespoons plus 1 teaspoon fish sauce

2 tablespoons water

2 tablespoons fresh lime juice

½ pound lean ground pork

1 pound lean ground lamb

1 carrot, peeled and grated

1 organic egg, beaten

For Scallions:

16 stalks scallions, trimmed

2 tablespoons coconut oil, melted

Salt, to taste

½ cup water

Directions:

Preheat the oven to 375 degrees F. Grease a baking dish.

In a food processor, add lemongrass, ginger, garlic, fresh herbs, fish sauce, water and lime juice and pulse till chopped finely.

Transfer the mixture into a bowl with remaining ingredients and mix till well combined.

Make about 1-inch balls from mixture.

Arrange the balls into prepared baking dish in a single layer.

In another rimmed baking dish, arrange scallion stalks in a single layer.

Drizzle with coconut oil and sprinkle with salt.

Pour water in the baking dish 1nd with a foil paper cover it tightly.

Bake the scallion for about 30 minutes.

Bake the meatballs for about 30-35 minutes.

Roasted Brussels Sprouts

Servings: 4

Preparation Time: 5 minutes

Cooking Time: 15 minutes

Total Time: 20 minutes

Ingredients

Sea salt .25 tsp.

Black pepper .25 tsp.

Brussel sprouts .75lbs. sliced in half length-wise

Coconut oil 5 T.

Directions

Ensure your oven is heated to 400F. Cut Brussels sprouts in half and place in a medium-sized bowl. Drizzle the coconut oil over the Brussels sprouts and then toss with the sea salt and black pepper until evenly coated.

Pour Brussels sprouts onto a baking sheet and make sure they are evenly spaced so that they will roast easily.

Place the sheet in the oven and let it cook approximately 10 minutes before stirring well and returning it to the oven for 10 minutes more. Season as desired They will keep in the fridge for 3-4 days, or in the freezer for 2-3 months.

Pork with Bell Pepper

This stir fry not only tastes wonderful but also is packed with nutritious benefits. Fresh lime juice intensifies the flavor of this stir fry.

Servings: 4

Preparation Time: 15 minutes

Cooking Time: 13 minutes

Ingredients:

1 tablespoon fresh ginger, chopped finely

4 garlic cloves, chopped finely

1 cup fresh cilantro, chopped and divided

¼ cup plus 1 tbsp olive oil, divided

1 pound tender pork, trimmed, sliced thinly

2 onions, sliced thinly

1 green bell pepper, seeded and sliced thinly

1 tablespoon fresh lime juice

Directions:

In a large bowl, mix together ginger, garlic, ½ cup of cilantro and ¼ cup of oil.

Add pork and coat with mixture generously.

Refrigerate to marinate for about 2 hours.

Heat a large skillet on medium-high heat.

Add pork mixture and stir fry for about 4-5 minutes.

Transfer the pork into a bowl.

In the same skillet, heat remaining oil on medium heat.

Add onion and sauté for about 3 minutes.

Stir in bell pepper and stir fry for about 3 minutes.

Stir in pork, lime juice and remaining cilantro and cook for about 2 minutes.

Serve hot.

Roasted Summer Squash

Servings: 4

Preparation Time: 5 minutes

Cooking Time: 30 minutes

Total Time: 35 minutes

Ingredients

Zucchini 3

Yellow squash 3

Kosher salt 5 T

Black pepper .5 T

Coconut oil 2 T

Directions

Ensure your oven is heated to 400F

Peel vegetables and cut into .25 inch thick slices.

Assemble vegetables on a baking sheet or pan and drizzle coconut oil on top. Sprinkle with seasoning as desired

Bake at 400F for 30 minutes.

Savory Baked Acorn Squash

Servings: 4

Preparation Time: 5 minutes

Cooking Time: 30 minutes

Total Time: 35 minutes

Ingredients

Acorn squash 1

Kosher salt as desired

Black pepper as desired

Coconut oil 2 tsp.

Smoked paprika as desired

Directions

Ensure your oven is heated to 425F.

Cut acorn squash in half lengthwise, then cut halves into quarters lengthwise. Scoop out seeds and discard.

Place the squash on baking sheet and drizzle coconut oil over the top of each quarter. Scatter with the smoked paprika, salt, and pepper and bake in the oven for 30 minutes.

Pork with Pineapple

A wonderfully delicious recipe which will surely impress a meat lover... Pineapple compliments pork tenderloin in a wonderful way.

Servings: 4

Preparation Time: 15 minutes

Cooking Time: 14 minutes

Ingredients:

2 tablespoons coconut oil

1½ pound pork tenderloin, trimmed and cut into bite-sized pieces

1 onion, chopped

2 minced garlic cloves

1 (1-inch) piece fresh ginger, minced

20-ounce pineapple, cut into chunks

1 large red bell pepper, seeded and chopped

¼ cup fresh pineapple juice

¼ cup coconut aminos

Salt and freshly ground black pepper, to taste

Directions:

In a large skillet, melt coconut oil on high heat.

Add pork and stir fry for about 4-5 minutes.

Transfer the pork into a bowl.

In the same skillet, heat remaining oil on medium heat.

Add onion, garlic and ginger and sauté for about 2 minutes.

Stir in pineapple and bell pepper and stir fry for about 3 minutes.

Stir in pork, pineapple juice and coconut aminos and cook for about 3-4 minutes.

Serve hot.

Caraway Pork Mix

Preparation time: ten mins

Cooking time: 40 minutes

Servings: 6

Ingredients:

2 pounds pork meat, boneless and cubed

2 yellow onions, chopped

1 tablespoon extra-virgin extra virgin olive oil

1 garlic cloves, minced

3 cups low-sodium chicken stock

2 tablespoons sweet paprika

1 teaspoon caraway seeds

Black pepper towards taste

2 tablespoons parsley, chopped

Directions:

Heat up a pot while using the oil over medium heat, add pork and brown it for 10 minutes.

Add onions, garlic, stock, caraway seeds, paprika and pepper, provide your boil, reduce temperature, cover and cook for half an hour.

Add parsley, toss, divide into bowls and serve.

Enjoy!

Nutrition Values: calories 310, fat 4, fiber 4, carbs 13, protein 15

Roasted Mixed Olives

Preparation and Cooking Time 40 minutes

Servings: 6

Ingredients:

Black olives, pitted: 1 cup

Kalamata olives, pitted: 1 cup

Green olives, stuffed with almonds and garlic: 1 cup

Garlic cloves, peeled: 10

Olive oil: ¼ cup

Herbes de Provence: 1 tablespoon

Lemon zest, grated: 1 teaspoon

Ground black pepper: to taste

Chopped thyme, for serving: ½ teaspoon

Directions:

Set oven to 425 0F and let preheat.

In the meantime, place all olives on a baking sheet lined with parchment paper, then add garlic and herbes de Provence, drizzle with oil and toss until coated.

Place the baking sheet into the oven and bake for 10 minutes.

Then add olives and continue baking for 20 minutes, stirring halfway through.

When done, divide olives evenly between serving plates, season with black pepper, sprinkle with lemon zest and thyme and toss until evenly coated.

Serve immediately.

Nutrition Values:

Calories: 189, Fat: 13, Fiber: 5, Carbs: 4, Protein: 5

Rolls of Sausage Pizzas

Preparation Time: 40 minutes

Servings: 6

Ingredients:

Pizza sauce, ¼ cup.

Shredded mozzarella cheese, 2 cup.

Cooked sausage, ½ cup.

Salt.

Pizza seasoning, 1 tsp.

Chopped onion, 2 tbsps.

Black pepper.

Chopped red and green bell peppers, ¼ cup.

Chopped tomato,

Directions:

Line a baking sheet. Grease it slightly. Over the sheet, spread mozzarella cheese and top with sprinkles of pizza seasoning. Set in an oven preheated to 400 0F and bake until done for 20 minutes.

Remove the pizza crust from the oven. Spread it with tomatoes, sausage, bell peppers and onion. Top with tomato sauce drizzling.

Take back to the oven and bake for another 10 minutes.

Remove the pizza from oven and allow to cool. Slice into 6 equal parts and roll. Enjoy your lunch.

Nutrition :

calories: 117, fiber: 1, carbs: 2, fat: 7, protein: 11

Lamb Burgers with Avocado Dip

A winner and delicious burger recipe for whole family… These burgers are great when with smooth and silky textured avocado dip.

Servings: 4-6

Preparation Time: 20 minutes

Cooking Time: 10 minutes

Ingredients:

For Burgers:

1 (2-inch) piece fresh ginger, grated

1 pound lean ground lamb

1 medium onion, grated

2 minced garlic cloves

1 bunch fresh mint leaves, chopped finely

2 teaspoons ground coriander

2 teaspoons ground cumin

½ teaspoon ground allspice

½ teaspoon ground cinnamon

Salt and freshly ground black pepper, to taste

1 tbsp olive oil

For Dip:

3 small cucumbers, peeled and grated

1 avocado, peeled, pitted and chopped

½ of garlic clove, crushed

2 tablespoons fresh lemon juice

2 tablespoons olive oil

2 tablespoons fresh dill, chopped finely

2 tablespoons chives, chopped finely

Salt and freshly ground black pepper, to taste

Directions:

Preheat the broiler of oven. Lightly, grease a broiler pan.

For burgers in a large bowl, squeeze the juice of ginger.

Add remaining ingredients and mix till well combined.

Make equal sized burgers from the mixture.

Arrange the burgers in broiler pan and broil for about 5 minutes per side.

Meanwhile for dip squeeze the cucumbers juice in a bowl.

In a food processor, add avocado, garlic, lemon juice and oil and pulse till smooth.

Transfer the avocado mixture in a bowl.

Add remaining ingredients and stir to combine.

Serve the burgers with avocado dip.

Mustard Pork Chops

Preparation time: ten mins

Cooking time: twenty minutes

Servings: 6

Ingredients:

2 pork chops

¼ cup organic essential olive oil

2 yellow onions, sliced

2 garlic cloves, minced

2 teaspoons mustard

1 teaspoon sweet paprika

Black pepper towards taste

½ teaspoon oregano, dried

Directions:

In a tiny bowl, mix oil with garlic, mustard, paprika, black pepper, and oregano and whisk well.

Add the pork chops, toss well leave aside to 10 mins.

Place the meat for the preheated grill over medium-high heat and cook for 10 minutes on both sides.

Divide pork chops between plates and serve employing a side salad.

Enjoy!

Nutrition Values: calories 314, fat 4, fiber 4, carbs 7, protein 17

Greek Mixed Roasted Vegetables

Servings: 4

Preparation Time: 15 minutes

Cooking Time: 45 minutes

Total Time: 60 minutes

Ingredients- Vegetables

1 eggplant peeled and diced .75-inch

Black pepper as desired

Kosher sea salt as desired

Extra virgin olive oil 2 T

Garlic 2 cloves minced

Onion 1 peeled, diced 1-inch

Bell pepper 2 red, yellow, diced, 1-inch

Ingredients- Dressing

Coconut oil .25 c

Lemon juice .3 c squeezed fresh

Black pepper as desired

Kosher sea salt as desired

Basil 15 leaves

Scallions 4 minced

Directions

Ensure your oven is heated to 425F.

One a sheet pan, combine the garlic, onion, yellow bell pepper, red bell pepper, and eggplant before seasoning using the pepper, salt, and coconut oil.

Add the pan to the oven and let it cook for 40 minutes, using a spatula to flip everything after 20 minutes.

As the vegetables are cooking, combine the pepper, salt, coconut oil, and lemon juice together in a small bowl, add the results to the vegetables as soon as they are ready.

Let the pan cool completely before adding in the basil, feta, and scallions. Season prior to serving.

Pork and Lentils Soup

Preparation time: ten mins

Cooking time: an hour and 5 minutes

Servings: 6

Ingredients:

1 small yellow onion, chopped

1 tablespoon olive oil

1 and ½ teaspoons basil, chopped

1 and ½ teaspoons ginger, grated

3 garlic cloves, chopped

Black pepper for the taste

1 carrot, chopped

1 pound pork chops, boneless and cubed

3 ounces brown lentils, rinsed

3 cups low sodium chicken stock

2 tablespoons tomato paste

2 tablespoons lime juice

Directions:

Heat up a pot with all the current oil over medium heat, add garlic, onion, basil, ginger, carrots and black pepper, stir and cook for 10 mins.

Add the pork and brown for 5 minutes more.

Add lentils, tomato paste and stock, bring with a boil, cover pot and simmer for 50 minutes.

Add lime juice, toss, ladle into bowls and serve.

Enjoy!

Nutrition Values: calories 273, fat 4, fiber 6, carbs 12, protein 16

Pork and Veggies Stew

Preparation time: 10 mins

Cooking time: 60 minutes and 10 minutes

Servings: 4

Ingredients:

½ cup low-sodium chicken stock

1 tablespoon ginger, grated

1 teaspoon coriander, ground

2 teaspoons cumin, ground

Black pepper for that taste

2 and ½ pounds pork butt, cubed

28 ounces canned tomatoes, no-salt-added, drained and chopped

4 ounces carrots, chopped

1 red onion, cut into wedges

4 garlic cloves, minced

15 ounces canned chickpeas, no-salt-added, drained and rinsed

1   tablespoon cilantro, chopped

Directions:

Heat up a pot over medium heat, add pork cubes and brown the crooks to minutes.

Add ginger, coriander, cumin, black pepper, onion, carrots and garlic, stir and cook for 5 minutes more.

Add the stock, the tomatoes also since the chickpeas, toss, bring to a simmer, cover the pot and cook for an hour.

Add cilantro, stir, divide into bowls and serve.

Enjoy!

Nutrition Values: calories 256, fat 6, fiber 8, carbs 12, protein 24

Pork and Snow Peas Salad

Preparation time: ten mins

Cooking time: 0 minutes

Servings: 4

Ingredients:

1 red chili, chopped

2 tablespoons balsamic vinegar

1/3 cup coconut aminos

1 tablespoon lime juice

1 teaspoon extra virgin olive oil

4 ounces mixed salad greens

4 ounces snow peas, blanched

1 red bell pepper, sliced

4 ounces pork, cooked and cut into thin strips

Directions:

In a salad bowl, mix greens with peas, bell pepper and pork..

Add the chili, vinegar, aminos, lime juice and oil, toss well and serve.

Enjoy!

Nutrition Values: calories 235, fat 4, fiber 4, carbs 12, protein 17

Pork and Beans Stew

Preparation time: twenty roughly minutes

Cooking time: 1 hour and ten mins

Servings: 4

Ingredients:

2 pounds pork butt, trimmed and cubed

1 and ½ tablespoons essential extra virgin olive oil

2 eggplants, chopped

1 yellow onion, chopped

1 red bell pepper, chopped

3 garlic cloves, minced

1 tablespoon thyme, dried

2 teaspoons sage, dried

4 ounces canned white beans, no-salt-added, drained and rinsed

1 cup low-sodium chicken stock

12 ounces zucchinis, chopped

2 tablespoons tomato paste

Directions:

Heat up a pot with all the oil over medium-high heat, add pork and brown for 5 minutes.

Add the onion, garlic, thyme, sage, bell pepper and eggplants, toss and cook for 5 minutes more.

Add beans, stock and tomato paste, toss, bring to a simmer, cover the pot and cook for 50 minutes.

Add the zucchinis, toss, cook for ten mins more, divide into bowls and serve.

Enjoy!

Nutrition Values: calories 310, fat 3, fiber 5, carbs 12, protein 22

Spiced Pork

One of the absolute delicious dish of spiced pork...
Slow cooking helps to infuse the spice flavors in pork
very nicely.

Servings: 6

Preparation Time: 15 minutes

Cooking Time: 1 hour 52 minutes

Ingredients:

1 (2-inch) piece fresh ginger, chopped

5-10 garlic cloves, chopped

1 teaspoon ground cumin

½ teaspoon ground turmeric

1 tablespoon hot paprika

1 tablespoon red pepper flakes

Salt, to taste

2 tablespoons cider vinegar

2 pounds pork shoulder, trimmed and cubed into
1½-inch size

2 cups hot water, divided

1 (1-inch wide) ball tamarind pulp

¼ cup olive oil

1 teaspoon black mustard seeds, crushed

4 green cardamoms

5 whole cloves

1 (3-inch) cinnamon stick

1 cup onion, chopped finely

1 large red bell pepper, seeded and chopped

Directions:

In a food processor, add ginger, garlic, cumin, turmeric, paprika, red pepper flakes, salt and cider vinegar and pulse till smooth.

Transfer the mixture into a large bowl.

Add pork and coat with mixture generously.

Keep aside, covered for about 1 hour at room temperature.

In a bowl, add 1 cup of hot water and tamarind and keep aside till water becomes cool.

With your hands, crush the tamarind to extract the pulp.

Add remaining cup of hot water and mix till well combined.

Through a fine sieve, strain the tamarind juice in a bowl.

In a large skillet, heat oil on medium-high heat.

Add mustard seeds, green cardamoms, cloves and cinnamon stick and sauté for about 4 minutes.

Add onion and sauté for about 5 minutes.

Add pork and stir fry for about 6 minutes.

Stir in tamarind juice and bring to a boil.

Reduce the heat to medium-low and simmer 1½ hours.

Stir in bell pepper and cook for about 7 minutes.

Pork Chili

A great bowl of healthy chili with an amazing addition of bokchoy. This healthy chili is tasty, spicy and refreshing at the same time.

Servings: 8

Preparation Time: 15 minutes

Cooking Time: 1 hour

Ingredients:

2 tablespoons extra-virgin olive oil

2 pound ground pork

1 medium red bell pepper, seeded and chopped

1 medium onion, chopped

5 garlic cloves, chopped finely

1 (2-inch) piece of hot pepper, minced

1 tablespoon ground cumin

1 teaspoon ground turmeric

3 tablespoon chili powder

½ teaspoon chipotle chili powder

Salt and freshly ground black pepper, to taste

1 cup chicken broth

1 (28-ounce) can fire-roasted crushed tomatoes

2 medium bokchoy heads, sliced

1 avocado, peeled, pitted and chopped

Directions:

In a large pan, heat oil on medium heat.

Add pork and stir fry for about 5 minutes.

Add bell pepper, onion, garlic, hot pepper and spices and stir fry for about 5 minutes.

Add broth and tomatoes and bring to a boil.

Stir in bokchoy and cook, covered for about 20 minutes.

Uncover and cook for about 20-30 minutes.

Serve hot with the topping of avocado.

Ground Pork with Water Chestnuts

This recipe is an easy way to prepare weeknight meal with a healthy touch... This recipe prepares a flavor packed meal.

Servings: 4

Preparation Time: 15 minutes

Cooking Time: 12 minutes

Ingredients:

1 tablespoon plus 1 teaspoon coconut oil

1 tablespoon fresh ginger, minced

1 bunch scallion (white and green parts separated), chopped

1 pound lean ground pork

Salt, to taste

1 tablespoon 5-spice powder

1 (18-ounce) can water chestnuts, drained and chopped

1 tablespoon organic honey

2 tablespoons fresh lime juice

Directions:

In a large heavy bottomed skillet, heat oil on high heat.

Add ginger and scallion whites and sauté for about ½-1½ minutes.

Add pork and cook for about 4-5 minutes.

Drain the excess fat from skillet.

Add salt and 5-spice powder and cook for about 2-3 minutes.

Add scallion greens and remaining ingredients and cook, stirring continuously for about 1-2 minutes.

Nutrition Values:

Calories: 520

Fat: 30g

Sat Fat: 6g

Carbohydrates: 37g

Fiber: 4g

Sugar: 9g

Protein: 25g

Sodium: 950mg

Glazed Pork chops with Peach

One of an easy and impressive way to enjoy pork and fresh peach in a delicious glaze... This sweet and spicy glaze makes pork super delicious.

Servings: 2

Preparation Time: 15 minutes

Cooking Time: 16 minutes

Ingredients:

2 boneless pork chops

Salt and freshly ground black pepper, to taste

1 ripe yellow peach, peeled, pitted, chopped and divided

1 tbsp olive oil

2 tablespoons shallot, minced

2 tablespoons garlic, minced

2 tablespoons fresh ginger, minced

1 tablespoon organic honey

1 tablespoon balsamic vinegar

1 tablespoon coconut aminos

¼ teaspoon red pepper flakes, crushed

¼ cup water

Directions:

Sprinkle the pork chops with salt and black pepper generously.

In a blender, add half of peach and pulse till a puree forms.

Reserve remaining peach.

In a skillet, heat oil on medium heat.

Add shallots and sauté for about 1-2 minutes.

Add garlic and ginger and sauté for about 1 minute.

Add remaining ingredients and reduce the heat to medium-low.

Bring to a boil and simmer for about 4-5 minutes or till a sticky glaze forms.

Remove from heat and reserve 1/3 of the glaze and keep aside.

Coat the chops with remaining glaze.

Heat a nonstick skillet on medium-high heat.

Add chops and sear for about 4 minutes from both sides.

Transfer the chops in a plate and coat with the remaining glaze evenly.

Top with reserved chopped peach and serve.

Pork chops in Creamy Sauce

Pork chops with extra twist of delish flavors... This special and easy technique of coconut sauce gives extra flavor and texture to pork chops.

Servings: 4

Preparation Time: 15 minutes

Cooking Time: 14 minutes

Ingredients:

2 garlic cloves, chopped

1 small jalapeño pepper, chopped

¼ cup fresh cilantro leaves

1½ teaspoons ground turmeric, divided

1 tablespoon fish sauce

2 tablespoons fresh lime juice

1 (13½-ounce) can coconut milk

4 (½-inch thick) pork chops

Salt, to taste

1 tablespoon coconut oil

1 shallot, chopped finely

Directions:

In a blender, add garlic, jalapeño pepper, cilantro, 1 teaspoon of ground turmeric, fish sauce, lime juice and coconut milk and pulse till smooth.

Sprinkle the pork with salt and remaining turmeric evenly.

In a skillet, melt butter on medium-high heat.

Add shallots and sauté for about 1 minute.

Add chops and cook for about 2 minutes per side.

Transfer the chops in a bowl.

Add coconut mixture and bring to a boil.

Reduce the heat to medium and simmer, stirring occasionally for about 5 minutes.

Stir in pork chops and cook for about 3-4 minutes.

Serve hot.

Baked Pork & Mushroom Meatballs

A healthy, hearty and tasty recipe of meatballs....
Fresh herbs add a really refreshing and aromatic
touch in these baked meatballs.

Servings: 6

Preparation Time: 15 minutes

Cooking Time: 15 minutes

Ingredients:

1 pound lean ground pork

1 organic egg white, beaten

4 fresh shiitake mushrooms, stemmed and minced

1 tablespoon fresh parsley, minced

1 tablespoon fresh basil leaves, minced

1 tablespoon fresh mint leaves, minced

2 teaspoons fresh lemon zest, grated finely

1½ teaspoons fresh ginger, grated finely

Salt and freshly ground black pepper, to taste

Directions:

Preheat the oven to 425 degrees F. Arrange the rack
in the center of oven.

Line a baking sheet with a parchment paper.

In a large bowl, add all ingredients and mix till well combined.

Make small equal-sized balls from mixture.

Arrange the balls onto prepared baking sheet in a single layer.

Bake for about 12-15 minutes or till done completely.

Chapter 12: Snacks Recipes

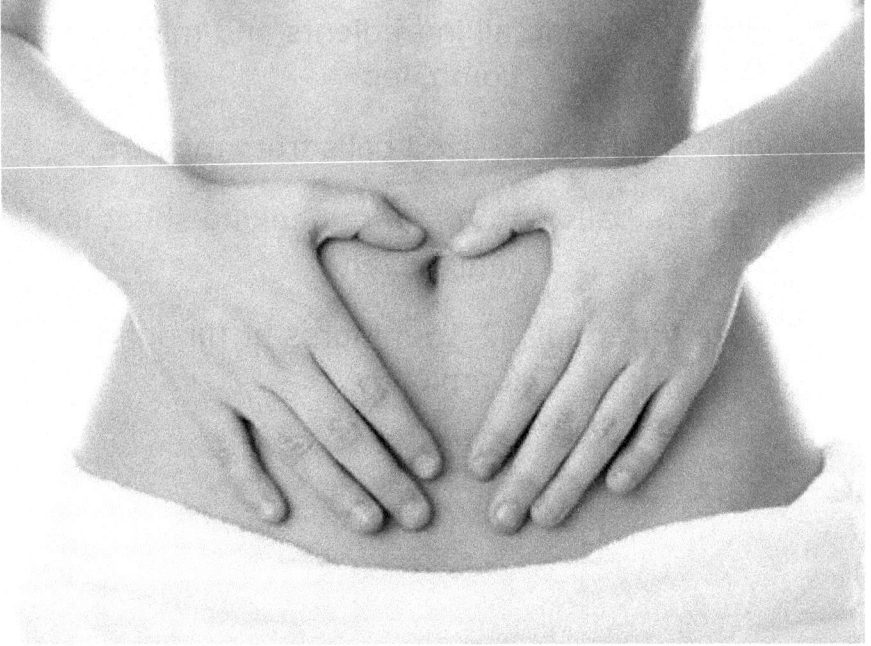

Chickpeas and Pepper Hummus

Preparation time: ten mins

Cooking time: 0 minutes

Servings: 4

Ingredients:

14 ounces canned chickpeas, no-salt-added, drained and rinsed

1 tablespoon sesame paste

2 roasted red peppers, chopped

Juice of ½ lemon

4 walnuts, chopped

Directions:

In your blender, combine the chickpeas with all the sesame paste, red peppers, lemon juice and walnuts, pulse well, divide into bowls and serve as as being a snack.

Enjoy!

Nutrition Values: calories 231, fat 12, fiber 6, carbs 15, protein 14

Lemony Chickpeas Dip

Preparation time: 10 mins

Cooking time: 0 minutes

Servings: 4

Ingredients:

14 ounces canned chickpeas, drained, no-salt-added, rinsed

Zest of merely one lemon, grated

Juice of a single lemon

1 tablespoon olive oil

4 tablespoons pine nuts

½ cup coriander, chopped

Directions:

In a blender, combine the chickpeas with lemon zest, freshly squeezed lemon juice, coriander and oil, pulse well, divide into small bowls, sprinkle pine nuts at the pinnacle and serve as a conference dip.

Enjoy!

Nutrition Values: calories 200, fat 12, fiber 4, carbs 9, protein 7

Chili Nuts

Preparation time: 10 minutes

Cooking time: 10 mins

Servings: 4

Ingredients:

½ teaspoon chili flakes

1 egg white

½ teaspoon curry powder

½ teaspoon ginger powder

4 tablespoons coconut sugar

A pinch of cayenne

14 ounces mixed nuts

Directions:

In a bowl, combine the egg white with all the chili flakes, curry powder, curry powder, ginger powder, coconut sugar and cayenne and whisk well.

Add the nuts, toss well, spread them having a lined baking sheet, introduce within the oven and bake at 400 degrees F for ten mins.

Divide the nuts into bowls and serve as a snack.

Enjoy!

Nutrition Values: calories 234, fat 12, fiber 5, carbs 14, protein 7

Protein Bars

Preparation time: ten mins

Cooking time: 0 minutes

Servings: 4

Ingredients:

4 ounces apricots, dried

2 ounces water

2 tablespoons rolled oats

1 tablespoon sunflower seeds

2 tablespoons coconut, shredded

1 tablespoon sesame seeds

1 tablespoon cranberries

3 tablespoons hemp seeds

1 tablespoon chia seeds

Directions:

In your food processor, combine the apricots while using water along with all the oats, pulse well, transfer for your bowl, add coconut, sunflower seeds, sesame seeds, cranberries, hemp and chia seeds and stir prior to getting a paste.

Roll this inside a log, wrap, cool inside fridge, slice and serve as a snack.

Enjoy!

Nutrition Values: calories 100, fat 3, fiber 4, carbs 8, protein 5

Eggplant, Olives and Basil Salad

Preparation Time: 15 minutes

Servings 4

Ingredients:

Tomatoes, chopped: 1 ½ cups

Eggplant, cubed: 3 cups

Capers: 2 teaspoons

Green olives, pitted and sliced: 6 ounces

Minced garlic: 2 teaspoons

Salt: ½ teaspoon

Ground black pepper: ¼ teaspoon

Chopped basil: 1 tablespoon

Olive oil: 2 teaspoons

Balsamic vinegar: 2 teaspoons

Directions:

Place a medium skillet pan over medium-high heat, add oil and when hot, add eggplant pieces and cook for 5 minutes.

Then add remaining ingredients, stir well and cook for 5 minutes.

When done, remove the pan from heat and let cool for 5 minutes.

Then divide salad evenly between small cups and serve as an appetizer.

Nutrition Values:

calories: 199, fat: 6, fiber: 5, carbs: 7, protein: 7

Fresh Tomato, Onion and Jalapeno Pepper Salsa

Preparation Time: 5 minutes

Servings 4

Ingredients:

Cherry tomatoes, halved: 2 cups

Red onion, peeled and chopped: ¼ cup

Jalapeno pepper, chopped: 1

Minced garlic: ½ teaspoon

Chopped cilantro: 2 tablespoons

Salt: ¼ teaspoon

Ground black pepper: ¼ teaspoon

Lime juice: 2 tablespoons

Directions:

Place all the ingredients for salsa in a medium bowl and stir until combined.

Serve straight away as a snack.

Nutrition Values:

calories: 87, fat: 1, fiber: 2, carbs: 7, protein: 5

Fresh Veggie Bars

Preparation Time: 40 minutes

Servings: 18

Ingredients:

Egg-1

Broccoli florets-2 cups

Cheddar cheese-1/3 cup (grated)

Onion-¼ cup (peeled and chopped)

Cauliflower rice-½ cup

Fresh parsley-2 tablespoons (chopped)

Olive oil-A drizzle (for greasing)

Salt and black pepper-to taste (ground)

Directions:

Warm up a saucepan with water over medium heat

Stir into the broccoli and let it simmer for a minute.

Strain and finely chop it to put into a bowl.

Mix in the egg, cheddar cheese, cauliflower rice, salt, pepper, parsley, and mix.

Give them the shape of bars by using the mixture on your hands.

Put them on a greased baking sheet.

Keep it in an oven at 400ºF and bake for 20 minutes.

Settle the prepared dish on a platter to serve.

Nutrition Values:

Calories: 19, Fat: 1, Fiber: 3, Carbs: 3, Protein: 3

Green Beans And Avocado with Chopped Cilantro

Preparation Time: 15 minutes

Servings: 4

Ingredients:

Avocados: 2; pitted and peeled

green beans - 2/3 pound, trimmed

scallions - 5, chopped.

olive oil - 3 tablespoons

A handful cilantro, chopped.

Salt and black pepper to the taste.

Directions:

Heat up a pan containing oil on a medium-high heat source; then add green beans and stir gently. Cook this mixture for about 4 minutes

Add salt and pepper to the pan; and stir gently, then remove the heat and move to a clean bowl.

Mix the avocados with salt and pepper and mash with a fork inside a clean bowl.

Then add onions and stir properly.

Add this over green beans, then toss to ensure it is well coated.

Finally, serve with some chopped cilantro on top.

Nutrition :

Calories:- 200; Fat : 5; Fiber : 3; Carbs : 4; Protein : 6

Italian Pizza Dip

Preparation Time: 30 minutes

Servings: 4

Ingredients:

Italian seasoning, ½ tsp.

Black pepper

Mozzarella cheese, ½ cup.

Chopped green bell pepper, 1 tbsp.

Sour cream, ¼ cup.

Salt

Grated Parmesan cheese, ¼ cup.

Tomato sauce, ½ cup.

Mayonnaise, ¼ cup.

Softened cream cheese, 4 oz.

Chopped pepperoni slices, 6

Chopped black olives, 4

Directions:

Gently stir together pepper, sour cream, cream cheese, mayonnaise, mozzarella cheese, and salt in a big bowl

Put the mixture into four ramekins then top with tomato sauce, parmesan cheese, then bell pepper, pepperoni, Italian seasoning, and black olives

Set your oven for 20 minutes at 350oF

Allow to bake

Enjoy the meal warm.

Nutrition Values:

Calories: 284, Fat: 24, Fiber: 1, Carbs: 5, Protein: 6

Jalapeno Cheesy Balls

Preparation Time: 10 minutes

Servings: 2

Ingredients:

Cream cheese, 3 oz.

Garlic powder, ¼ tsp.

Onion powder, ¼ tsp.

Black pepper

Chopped jalapeno peppers, 2

Salt

Dried parsley, ½ tsp.

Cooked and crumbled bacon slices, 3

Directions:

Set the mixing bowl in position to combine garlic powder, bacon, seasonings, parsley, and onion with the jalapeno peppers

Shape the mixture into balls

Set the balls on a flat plate to take as a cold appetizer

Nutrition Values:

Calories: 200, Fat: 5, Fiber: 4, Carbs: 12, Protein: 6

Keto Veggie Noodles: Side Dish

Preparation Time: 30 minutes

Servings: 6

Ingredients:

Zucchini - 1, cut with a spiralizer

summer squash - 1, cut with a spiralizer

yellow, orange and red bell peppers - 6 ounces; cut into thin strips

bacon fat - 4 tablespoons

garlic cloves - 3, minced

carrot - 1, cut with a spiralizer

sweet potato - 1, cut with a spiralizer

red onion - 4 ounces, chopped.

Salt and black pepper to the taste.

Directions:

Arrange zucchini noodles neatly on a lined baking sheet.

Then add squash, carrot, sweet potato, onion and all bell peppers

Sprinkle a pinch of salt, pepper and garlic and toss to coat.

Then add bacon fat, toss again all noodles.

Move to an oven set at a temperature of 400 oF and bake for about 20 minutes

Move to clean plates. Serve immediately as a keto side dish.

Nutrition :

Calories:- 50; Fat : 1; Fiber : 1; Carbs : 6; Protein : 2

Minty Zucchini Rolls

Preparation Time: 20 minutes

Servings: 24

Ingredients:

Chopped basil, ¼ cup.

Sliced zucchinis, 3

Ricotta cheese, 1 1/3 cup.

Salt

Chopped mint, 2 tbsps.

Black pepper

Basil leaves, 24

Olive oil, 2 tbsps.

Directions:

Prepare the baking tray by lining well.

Add the zucchini slices then splash the oil and the seasonings on it

Set the oven for 10 minutes at 3750F, allow to bake

Meanwhile, set the mixing bowl in position to stir together chopped basil, ricotta, seasonings, and mint.

Divide the mixture on the zucchini slices as you roll

Set the rolls on a flat plate

Enjoy

Nutrition Values:

Calories: 172, Fat: 3, Fiber: 4, Carbs: 9, Protein: 4

Sesame Zucchini Spread

Preparation Time: 16 minutes

Servings: 4

Ingredients:

Lemon juice, ½ cup.

Veggie stock, 3 tbsps.

Olive oil, ¼ cup.

Salt

Chopped zucchinis, 4 cup.

Black pepper

Minced garlic cloves, 4

Sesame seeds paste, ¾ cup.

Directions:

Set your pan over medium-high heat with half of the oil to cook the garlic and zucchini for two minutes

Stir in the seasonings and stock to cook for four minutes

Move the zucchinis to the blender with the remaining oil, lemon juice, and sesame seeds paste to process until smooth.

Set the mixture in bowls to serve

Enjoy.

Nutrition Values:

Calories: 140, Fat: 5, Fiber: 3, Carbs: 6, Protein: 7

Shrimp Salad with Tomato and Radish

Preparation Time: 10 minutes

Servings 8

Ingredients:

Shrimp, cooked, peeled and deveined: 1 pound

Medium white onion, chopped: ¼ cup

Tomato, cubed: 1

Radishes, chopped: 4

Minced jalapeno: 1 ½ teaspoon

Salt: ¼ teaspoon

Ground black pepper: ¼ teaspoon

Lime juice: 2 tablespoons

Chopped cilantro: ¼ cup

Directions:

Place all the ingredients for the salad in a medium bowl and stir until combined.

Serve salad straightaway as an appetizer.

Nutrition Values:

calories: 90, fat: 1, fiber: 1, carbs: 2, protein: 6

Shrimp wrapped with prosciutto

Preparation Time: 30 minutes

Servings: 16

Ingredients:

Red wine, 1/3 cup.Chopped mint, 1 tbsp.

Erythritol, 2 tbsps.

Cooked shrimp, 10 oz.

Olive oil, 2 tbsps.

Blackberries, 1/3 cup.

Sliced prosciutto 11

Directions:

Have the shrimp well wrapped with prosciutto slices.

Arrange the wrapped shrimp in a baking sheet then sprinkle with olive oil

Set the oven for 15 minutes at 4250F then allow to bake.

In the meantime, heat the mashed blackberries over medium heat.

Stir in erythritol, mint, and wine.

Set the shrimp on a serving plate, top the blackberries sauce and enjoy.

Nutrition Values:

Calories: 89, Fat: 5, Fiber: 2, Carbs: 1, Protein: 11

Simple Tomato Tarts

Preparation Time: 1 hour 20 minutes

Servings: 12

Ingredients:

Salt

Olive oil, ¼ cup.

Black pepper

Sliced tomatoes, 2

For the base:

Coconut flour, 2 tbsps.

Psyllium husk, 1 tbsp.

Butter, 5 tbsps.

Almond flour, ½ cup.

Salt

For the filling:

Sliced onion, 1Chopped thyme, 3 tsps.

Olive oil, 2 tbsps.

Minced garlic, 2 tbsps.

Crumbled goats cheese, 3 oz.

Directions:

Season the tomato slices then align on a baking sheet then dazzle some olive oil.

Set your oven for 40 minutes at 4250F.

Allow to bake

On the other hand, combine cold butter, coconut flour, pepper, almond flour, salt, psyllium husk in a food processor to achieve a dough.

Divide dough into silicone cupcake molds, press.

Set the oven for 20 minutes at 3500F then allow to bake.

Once fully baked, remove from oven and reserve.

Remove the tomato slices from the oven and allow them to cool

Top the tomato slices on the cupcakes

Meanwhile, quick fry the onions in a pan over medium-high heat, for about four minutes.

Stir in thyme and garlic, for about one minute.

Spread mixture on top of tomato slices.

Sprinkle the goat cheese on top.

Set your oven for 5 minutes at 350 oF

Bake until the cheese melts away

Enjoy

Nutrition Values:

Calories: 125, Fat: 17, Fiber: 1, Carbs: 1, Protein: 9

Special Tomato AndBocconcini: Side Dish

Preparation Time: 6 minutes

Servings: 4

Ingredients:

babybocconcini - 8 ounces, drain and torn

basil leaves - 1 cup, roughly chopped.

Tomatoes - 20 ounces, cut in wedges

stevia - 1 teaspoon

garlic clove - 1, finely minced

extra virgin olive oil - 2 tablespoons

balsamic vinegar - 1½ tablespoons

Salt and black pepper to the taste.

Directions:

Mix stevia with vinegar, garlic, oil, salt and pepper in a bowl and whisk very well.

Add bocconcini with tomato and basil to a clean salad and mix.

Add dressing, toss to keep well coated

Serve immediately as a keto side dish.

Nutrition Values:

Calories:- 100; Fat : 2; Fiber : 2; Carbs : 1; Protein : 9

Stir-Fried Queso

Preparation Time: 20 minutes

Servings: 6

Ingredients:

Olive oil, 1 ½ tbsps.

Cubed Queso Blanco, 5 oz.

Chopped olives, 2 oz.

Red pepper flakes

Directions:

Set up the pan to heat the oil over medium-high heat to cook the Queso cubes

Turn the Queso cubes using a spatula then sprinkle with olives

Allow the cubes to cook more for 5 minutes then turn again to sprinkle with red pepper flake.

Allow to cook to a crispy texture.

Turn the cubes again to cook on the other side

Once cooked, set on the chopping board then slice into small pieces

Enjoy.

Nutrition Values:

Calories: 152, Fat: 18, Fiber: 3, Carbs: 6, Protein: 2

Potato Chips

Preparation time: ten mins

Cooking time: 30 minutes

Servings: 6

Ingredients:

2 gold potatoes, cut into thin rounds

1 tablespoon olive oil

2 teaspoons garlic, minced

Directions:

In a bowl, combine the french fries while using the oil along with the garlic, toss, spread more than a lined baking sheet, introduce inside the oven and bake at 400 degrees F for a half-hour.

Divide into bowls and serve.

Enjoy!

Nutrition Values: calories 200, fat 3, fiber 5, carbs 13, protein 6

Peach Dip

Preparation time: ten mins

Cooking time: 0 minutes

Servings: 2

Ingredients:

½ cup nonfat yogurt

1 cup peaches, chopped

A pinch of cinnamon powder

A pinch of nutmeg, ground

Directions:

In a bowl, combine the yogurt while using the peaches, cinnamon and nutmeg, whisk, divide into small bowls and serve being a snack.

Enjoy!

Nutrition Values: calories 165, fat 2, fiber 3, carbs 14, protein 13

Cereal Mix

Preparation time: 10 mins

Cooking time: 40 minutes

Servings: 6

Ingredients:

3 tablespoons extra virgin organic olive oil

1 teaspoon hot sauce

½ teaspoon garlic powder

½ teaspoon onion powder

½ teaspoon cumin, ground

A pinch of red pepper cayenne

3 cups rice cereal squares

1 cup cornflakes

½ cup pepitas

Directions:

In a bowl, combine the oil while using the hot sauce, garlic powder, onion powder, cumin, cayenne, rice cereal, cornflakes and pepitas, toss, spread on the lined baking sheet, introduce inside the oven and bake at 350 degrees F for 40 minutes.

Divide into bowls and serve as a snack.

Enjoy!

Nutrition Values: calories 199, fat 3, fiber 4, carbs 12, protein 5

Easy Tuna Cakes

Preparation Time: 18 minutes

Servings: 12

Ingredients:

A drizzle of olive oil

Medium eggs, 3

Dried parsley, 1 tsp.

Garlic powder, 1 tsp.

Salt

Chopped red onion, ½ cup.

Black pepper

Canned tuna, 15 oz.

Directions:

Set a mixing bowl in position to stir together parsley, seasonings, eggs, garlic powder, and onion then mold the mixture into patties.

Set a pan on fire with the oil to cook the cakes evenly over medium-high heat.

Set the patties on a serving platter and enjoy as an appetizer

Nutrition Values:

Calories: 160, Fat: 2, Fiber: 4, Carbs: 6, Protein: 6

Mushrooms Stuffed with shrimp mixture.

Preparation Time: 30 minutes

Servings: 5

Ingredients:

Cooked shrimp, 1 cup.

Garlic powder, 1 tsp.

Salt

Chopped onion, 1

Chopped white mushroom caps, 24 oz.

Black   pepper

Softened cream cheese, 4 oz.

Mayonnaise, ¼ cup.

Sour cream, ¼ cup.

Curry powder, 1 tsp.

Quesoblanco or Monterey Jack cheese, ½ cup.

Directions:

Set the mixing bowl in a working surface.

Whisk in onion, mayonnaise, shrimp, curry powder, Mexican cheese, Pepper, cream cheese, garlic powder, salt, and sour cream.

Fill the mushrooms with the combination and set on a baking tray

Set your oven for 20 minutes at 350oF, allow too bake

Enjoy the meal once fully baked

Nutrition Values:

Calories: 259, Fat: 18, Fiber: 9, Carbs: 17, Protein: 16

Oven-baked Crackers

Preparation Time: 25 minutes

Servings: 6

Ingredients:

Ghee, 3 tbsps.

Salt

Minced garlic clove, 1

Black pepper

Dried basil, ¼ tsp.

Baking powder, ½ tsp.

Basil pesto, 2 tbsps.

Almond flour, 1¼ cup.

Directions:

Set the mixing bowl in position to combine the almond flour, seasonings, basil pesto, baking powder, ghee, and the garlic to make a dough

Line the baking tray then set the dough on it.

Set the oven for 17 minutes at 3250F, allow to bake

Slice into medium crackers the moment they are cold then serve them as a snack.

Enjoy

Nutrition Values:

Calories: 200, Fat: 20, Fiber: 1, Carbs: 4, Protein: 7

Parmesan Spinach Balls

Preparation Time: 22 minutes

Servings: 30

Ingredients:

Whipping cream, 3 tbsps.

Grated Parmesan cheese, 1/3 cup.

Medium eggs, 2

Crumbled feta cheese, 1/3 c

Almond flour, 1 cup.

Spinach, 16 oz.

Salt

Melted butter, 4 tbsps.

Ground nutmeg, ¼ tsp.

Black pepper

Onion powder, 1 tbsp.

Garlic powder, 1 tsp.

Directions:

Plug in and set your food processor in position

Add in feta cheese, spinach, nutmeg, eggs, whipping cream, garlic powder, almond flour, pepper, butter, onion, and salt.

Process until smooth. Pour the mixture in a bowl to refrigerate in the freezer for 10 minutes.

Mold into 30 spinach balls and set them on a well-greased baking tray. Set your oven for 12 minutes at 350 0F, allow to bake thoroughly.

Allow the balls to cool and enjoy

Nutrition Values:

Calories: 40, Fat: 5, Fiber: 5, Carbs: 1, Protein: 7

Pecan with Maple syrup Bars

Preparation Time: 35 minutes

Servings: 12

Ingredients:

Maple syrup, ¼ cup.

Stevia, ¼ tsp.

Crushed pecans, toasted, 2 cup.

Almond flour, 1 cup.

Coconut oil, ½ cup.

Flaxseed meal, ½ cup.

Shredded coconut, ½ cup.

For the maple syrup:

Vanilla extract, ½ tsp.

Coconut oil, 2 ¼ tbsp.

Xanthan gum, ¼ tsp.

Erythritol, ¼ cup.

Water, ¾ cup.

Maple extract, 2 tsps.

Butter, 1 tbsp.

Directions:

Microwave 2¼ teaspoon coconut oil, butter, xanthan gum, in a heatproof bowl for about one minute.

Mix in maple, erythritol, vanilla extract, and water as you stir gently.

Microwave again for another one minute.

Meanwhile, combine coconut flour, flaxseed meal, and almond flour in another bowl as you stir gently.

Stir in the pecans then add coconut oil, ¼ cup maple syrup, and stevia.

Set the mixture in a baking sheet

Set your oven for 25 minutes at 3500F then allow to bake.

Allow cooling before slicing and serving.

Nutrition Values:

Calories: 313, Fat: 31, Fiber: 3, Carbs: 18, Protein: 7

Plum and Jalapeno Salad with Basil

Preparation Time: 10 minutes

Servings 6

Ingredients:

Plums, chopped: 1 cup

Chopped basil: 2 tablespoons

Jalapeno pepper, chopped: 1

Red onion, peeled and chopped: 2 tablespoons

Lime juice: 2 teaspoons

Salt: ½ teaspoon

Ground black pepper: ¼ teaspoon

Stevia: 2 tablespoons

Ground cumin: ½ teaspoon

Olive oil: 1 teaspoon

Directions:

Place all the ingredients for the salad in a medium bowl and stir until combined.

Place salad bowl in a refrigerator for 1 hour or until chilled and then serve as an appetizer.

Nutrition Values:

calories: 137, fat: 2, fiber: 2, carbs: 7, protein: 5

Seasoned Easy Fried Cabbage

Preparation Time: 25 minutes

Servings: 4

Ingredients:

green cabbage - 1½ pound, shredded

ghee - 5 ounces

A pinch of sweet paprika

Salt and black pepper to the taste.

Directions:

Add heat to a pan containing ghee over medium-high heat source.

Then pour some cabbage to the pan and cook for 15 minutes stirring frequently.

Then sprinkle a pinch of salt, pepper and paprika.

Stir gently, cook for another minute

Divide into different plates

Now you can serve

Nutrition :

Calories:- 200; Fat : 4; Fiber : 2; Carbs : 3; Protein : 7

Tasty Avocado Spread

Preparation Time: 1 minute

Servings: 4

Ingredients:

Stevia, ¼ tsp.

Halved avocados, 2

Juice of 2 limes

Coconut milk, 1 cup.

Chopped cilantro, ½ cup.

Zest of 2 limes

Directions:

Plug and switch on the blender in position.

Add in the stevia, avocados, lime juice, coconut milk, and cilantro, and lime zest to process until smooth.

Set into serving bowls to enjoy

Nutrition Values:

Calories: 190, Fat: 6, Fiber: 2, Carbs: 9, Protein: 6

Red Pepper Muffins

Preparation time: ten minutes

Cooking time: half an hour

Servings: 12

Ingredients:

1 and ¾ cups whole wheat grains flour

2 teaspoons baking powder

2 tablespoons coconut sugar

A pinch of black pepper

1 egg

¾ cup almond milk

2/3 cup roasted red pepper, chopped

½ cup low-fat mozzarella, shredded

Directions:

In a bowl, combine the flour with baking powder, coconut sugar, black pepper, egg, milk, red pepper and mozzarella, stir well, divide in a very lined muffin tray, introduce in the oven and bake at 400 degrees F for a half-hour.

Serve like a snack.

Enjoy!

Nutrition Values: calories 149, fat 4, fiber 2, carbs 14, protein 5

Nuts and Seeds Mix

Preparation time: 10 mins

Cooking time: 0 minutes

Servings: 6

Ingredients:

1 cup pecans

1 cup hazelnuts

1 cup almonds

¼ cup coconut, shredded

1 cup walnuts

½ cup papaya pieces, dried

½ cup dates, dried, pitted and chopped

½ cup sunflower seeds

½ cup pumpkin seeds

1 cup raisins

Directions:

In a bowl, combine the pecans with all the hazelnuts, almonds, coconut, walnuts, papaya, dates, sunflower seeds, pumpkin seeds and raisins, toss and serve as a snack.

Enjoy!

Nutrition Values: calories 188, fat 4, fiber 6, carbs 8, protein 6

Tortilla Chips

Preparation time: ten mins

Cooking time: 25 minutes

Servings: 6

Ingredients:

12 whole wheat grains grains tortillas, cut into 6 wedges each

2 tablespoons organic extra virgin olive oil

1 tablespoon chili powder

A pinch of cayenne

Directions:

Spread the tortillas for the lined baking sheet, add the oil, chili powder and cayenne, toss, introduce inside oven and bake at 350 degrees F for 25 minutes.

Divide into bowls and serve as as a side dish.

Enjoy!

Nutrition Values: calories 199, fat 3, fiber 4, carbs 12, protein 5

Kale Chips

Preparation time: ten mins

Cooking time: fifteen minutes

Servings: 8

Ingredients:

1 bunch kale leaves

1 tablespoon organic olive oil

1 teaspoon smoked paprika

A pinch of black pepper

Directions:

Spread the kale leaves over a baking sheet, add black pepper, oil and paprika, toss, introduce inside oven and bake at 350 degrees F for quarter-hour.

Divide into bowls and serve being a snack.

Enjoy!

Nutrition Values: calories 177, fat 2, fiber 4, carbs 13, protein 6

Pan-Fried Cheesy Sticks

Preparation Time: 1 hour 30 minutes

Servings: 16

Ingredients:

Black pepper

Mozzarella string cheese pieces, 8

Whisked eggs, 2

Italian seasoning, 1 tbsp.

Olive oil, ½ cup.

Grated Parmesan cheese, 1 cup.

Minced garlic clove, 1

Salt

Directions:

Set a medium mixing bowl on a clean working area.

Stir together salt, Italian seasoning, parmesan cheese, pepper, and garlic

In another mixing bowl, place the whisked eggs then coat the mozzarella sticks in egg mixture then cheese mixture.

Repeat the process twice to coat well then freeze for an hour.

After one hour, heat the oil in a pan over medium-high heat to fry the sticks to a golden color evenly

Set on a platter and enjoy

Nutrition Values:

Calories: 116, Fat: 14, Fiber: 0, Carbs: 8, Protein: 8

546. Pan-fried Italian Meatballs

Preparation Time: 16 minutes

Servings: 16

Ingredients:

Chopped basil, 2 tbsps.

Salt

Chopped sundried tomatoes, 2 tbsps.

Black pepper

Almond flour, ¼ cup.

Large egg, 1Ground turkey, 1 lb.

Shredded mozzarella cheese, ½ cup.

Garlic powder, ½ tsp.

Olive oil, 2 tbsps.

Directions:

Set your medium size mixing bowl in a clean working surface

Stir together the egg, ground turkey, garlic powder, pepper, basil, salt, mozzarella, almond flour, and sun-dried tomatoes

Mold the mixture into12 even meatballs

Set the pan over medium-high heat to melt the oil

Fry the meatballs in the oil until browned

Enjoy

Nutrition Values:

Calories: 81, Fat: 5, Fiber: 1, Carbs: 5, Protein: 5

Parmesan Basil Dip

Preparation Time: 5 minutes

Servings 10

Ingredients:

Chopped basil: 1 tablespoon

Minced garlic: ½ teaspoon

Lemon juice: 1 teaspoon

Basil pesto: 2 tablespoons

Avocado mayonnaise: 1 cup

Grated parmesan cheese: 1 tablespoon

Directions:

Place all the ingredients for the dip in a medium bowl and stir until combined.

Divide dip evenly between small bowls and serve.

Nutrition Values:

calories: 100, fat: 4, fiber: 2, carbs: 5, protein: 3

Parmesan Chicken Wings

Preparation Time: 34 minutes

Servings: 6

Ingredients:

Medium egg, 1 Black pepper

Italian seasoning, ½ tsp.

Butter, 2 tbsps.

Salt

Halved chicken wings, 6 lbs.

Grated Parmesan cheese, ½ cup.

Red pepper flakes, ¼ tsp.

Garlic powder, 1 tsp.

Directions:

Line the baking tray well and arrange the wings.

Set the oven for 17 minutes at 425 0F. Allow to bake.

Meanwhile, plug in and set the food processor in position.

Add in the Italian seasoning, butter, salt, garlic powder, cheese, red pepper flakes, egg, and pepper. Blend to mix well

Once the oven timer beeps, remove the wings and turn them.

Set the oven to broil

Allow the chicken wings to broil for 5 minutes

Remove the wings to coat with sauce over

Broil again for one minute.

Enjoy.

Nutrition Values:

Calories: 677, Fat: 51, Fiber: 0, Carbs: 1, Protein: 52

Chapter 13: Healthy and Delicious Beverages

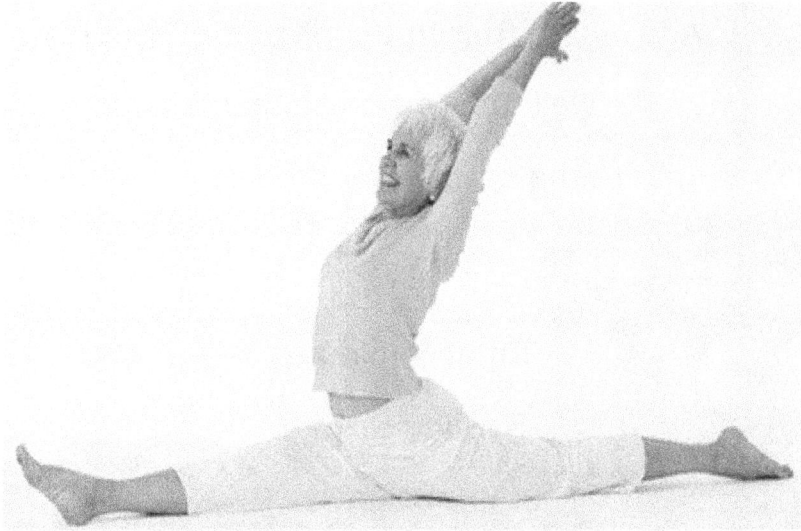

Citrus Flavored Water

Time: 20 minutes

Serving Size: 4

Ingredients:

I 1 cup of sliced lemons

I ½ cup of sliced limes

I 1 cup of sliced oranges

I 2 cups of diced watermelon

I 1 cup of sliced cucumbers

I A pitcher of cold water

Directions:

1. Add all the fruit to the pitcher of water.

2. Stir well to incorporate the flavors.

3. Refrigerate the mixture for several hours before serving.

Basil-Infused Tomato Water

Time: 5 minutes

Serving Size: 4

Ingredients:

l 1 diced red tomato

l 3 branches of crushed basil

l A pitcher of cold water

Directions:

1. Add the tomato and basil to the pitcher of water.

2. Stir well to incorporate the flavors.

3. Refrigerated for at least two hours to allow the fruit flavor to infuse the water. Strain and serve chilled. This can be refrigerated up to two days.

Refreshing Strawberry

Time: 5 minutes

Serving Size: 6

Ingredients:

I 1 cup stemmed and sliced strawberries

I 1 cup of sliced cucumbers I A pitcher of cold water

Directions:

1. Add all the fruit to the pitcher of water.

2. Stir well to incorporate the flavors.

3. Refrigerated for at least two hours to allow the fruit flavor to infuse the water.

Strain and serve chilled. This can be refrigerated up to two days.

Grapefruit Water

Time: 5 minutes

Serving Size: 6

Ingredients:

I 1 cup of fresh squeezed grapefruit juice

I A pitcher of cold water Directions:

4. Add the grapefruit juice to the water.

5. Refrigerate and serve chilled.

Black Lemon Iced Tea

Time: 5 minutes

Serving Size: 6

Ingredients:

I 6 cups water

I 3 black tea bags

I ½ cup of stevia

I ¼ cup orange juice

I ¼ cup lemon juice

I Fresh mint leaves

Directions:

1. Bring three cups of water to a boil over medium heat in a large saucepan. Remove from the heat and steep the tea bag for five minutes.

2. Remove the tea bags and discard.

3. Move the tea to a large pitcher and add the remaining ingredients.

4. Refrigerate and served chilled. Garnish with mint.

Raspberries Iced Tea

Time: 15 minutes

Serving Size: 8

Ingredients:

I 3 cups fresh raspberries

I ¼ cup of stevia I 1 tablespoon chopped fresh mint

I A pinch of baking soda

I 4 cups boiling water

I 2 green tea bags

Directions:

1. Combine raspberries and stevia in large bowl. Crush the mixture with wooden spoon.

2. Add the mint and baking soda. mix and set aside.

3. Steep the tea bags in boiling water. cover and let stand three minutes then remove and Discard the tea bags.

4. Pour green tea over raspberry mixture and let stand at room temperature for at least an hour. Strain the raspberry tea and served chilled.

Chamomile Orange Iced Tea

Time: 10 minutes

Serving Size: 8

Ingredients:

| 8 chamomile tea bags

| 12 cups of boiling water

| 1 cup of orange juice

| 4 teaspoons stevia

Directions:

1. Steep the tea bags in boiling water for five minutes.

2. Remove and discard the tea back and allow the tea to cool completely before adding the remaining ingredients. Stir to mix. 3. Refrigerate and serve chilled or with ice.

Mint Tea

Time: 10 minutes

Serving Size: 5

Ingredients:

| 5 cups of boiling water

| 2 green tea bags

| 6 mint leaves

| 4 teaspoons stevia

Directions:

1. Steep the tea bags in boiling water for five minutes.

2. Remove and discard the tea back and allow the tea to cool completely before adding the remaining ingredients. Stir to mix. 3. Strain and serve immediately. This can be refrigerated and served chilled.

Basil Ginger Tea

Time: 15 minutes

Serving Size: 2

Ingredients:

I 3 large basil leaves

I ½ teaspoon of finely grated ginger

I Boiled water

Directions:

1. Add all the ingredients to a teapot and brew until it reached your desired strength.

2. Sieve the basil and ginger, and serve

3. This beverage can be served cold by adding ice or refrigerating.

Green Veggie Juice

Time: 5 minutes

Serving Size: 2

Ingredients:

I 4 celery stalks

I ½ cup of diced cucumber

I 1 cup of diced pineapple

I ½ cup of diced green apple

I 1 cup of washed spinach

I 1 lemon

I ¼ cup of sliced ginger

Directions:

3. Add all the ingredients to a juicer and juice.

4.   Consume the juice immediately.

Pineapple Juice

Time: 10 minutes

Serving Size: 2

Ingredients:

I 2 cups of cubed pineapple

I 1 cup of water

I ½ inch of ginger

| ½ teaspoon of salt

| 3 basil leaves

| 1 tablespoon of lemon juice

Directions:

1. Add all the ingredients to a blender and blend until smooth.

2. Strain to remove solid bit and serve immediately. Can be served with ice.

CONCLUSION

Although the anti-inflammatory diet is generally good for health, it is especially suitable for treating some health problems. For example, the anti-inflammatory diet reduces the risk of heart disease, keeps existing heart problems under control, reduces blood pressure and triglycerides in the blood (natural fats formed by the combination of fatty acids and glycerol) and soothes hard rheumatic joints.

This diet aims to increase physical and mental health by recommending healthy, fat, fiber-rich fruits and vegetables, abundant water, and a limited amount of animal protein (excluding fish), providing a constant source of energy and reducing the risk of age-related diseases.

INTERMITTENT FASTING COOKBOOK OVER 50

A Beginner's Cookbook Guide with 60 Recipes for Rapid Weight Loss

Introduction:

Intermittent fasting is essentially a method of changing or exchanging your diet examples to ensure that you eat during various occasions in a day. Intermittent fasting works essentially by following a set eating less junk food plan. First, you eat regularly for the initial 5 days and afterward for the following 2 days you take in under 600 calories

Intermittent Fasting isn't tied in with starving yourself. It is essentially about abandoning nourishment for a brief timeframe period, then continuing your life regularly. Eating like a bunny all the time is a surefire way to tumble off your diet and damage your objectives. Eating like a hare part of the time, and practicing order and control is a powerful method to improve your weight loss endeavors and arrive at your objectives.

Intermittent fasting will give your body a little push with the capacity of consuming fat. Your body will abruptly figure out how to consume a lot of fat in a short measure of time. Intermittent refers to fasting; not eating anything and just drinking water for at least 24 hours. As incredible as this may appear, Intermittent fasting has been exceptionally effective for some people in helping them with getting thinner and feel better as a rule. It helps our bodies with copying fat rapidly severally.

Chapter: 1 Breakfast

1: Breakfast Oatmeal Cupcakes

These adjustable breakfast heated cereal cupcakes are incredible in a hurry fuel for those occasions when you have zero time in the first part of the day to set up a major feast. You can undoubtedly switch around the flavor by picking various flavors and add-ins for perpetual breakfast cupcake varieties.

This recipe makes preparing with stevia fun and simple. You can make these sound prepared cereal breakfast cups early and stash them in the cooler for a fast and filling breakfast.

Ingredients:

- 5 cups moved oats
- 1 tsp salt
- 2 1/2 cups over-ready crushed banana
- 5 tbsp unadulterated maple syrup, agave, or honey OR stevia comparable sum
- 2 1/3 cups water - Increase to 2/3 cups if utilizing stevia
- 2/3 cup smaller than usual chocolate chips, optional
- 1/4 cup + 1 tbsp coconut or veg oil (45g)
- Optional add-ins: cinnamon, chopped pecans, smashed coconut, ground flax or raw grain, raisins or other dried fruit, and so forth
- 2 1/2 tsp unadulterated vanilla concentrate

Method:

- Preheat stove to 380 F, and line 24-25 cupcake tins.
- In a large blending bowl, consolidate every dry ingredient and mix well overall.
- In a different bowl, consolidate and mix every single wet ingredient (counting banana).
- Blend wet into dry, then fill the cupcake liners and heat 21 minutes. I also prefer to then sear for 1-2 minutes, however, it's optional.
- These cereal cakes can be consumed right, or they can be frozen and warmed for a moment breakfast on a bustling day.

2: Raisin Oatmeal Muffins

Here is another incredible, without a wheat recipe. If you experience difficulty getting your children to have a sound breakfast, try this one. Expectation you and your family will appreciate these biscuits similarly as. These oats biscuits are produced using essential ingredients; such as ingredients you would have found in your grandma's washroom. However, being stacked with the supported energy of moved oats I have a little stunt that keeps them light and fleecy.

Ingredients:

- 1 cup whole wheat flour
- 1/3 cup sugar
- 2 teaspoons preparing powder

- 3/4 cup milk
- 1 egg
- 1/4 cup oil
- spread (genuine margarine) for the container
- 1/2 to 1 cup raisins
- 1 cup oats (moved breakfast oats), conventional sluggish (large) type

Method:

- Pre-heat a stove to 375°F.
- Spread a biscuit container or cupcake skillet.
- Spot the dry ingredients in a single bowl, and the wet ingredients in an alternate bowl.
- Blend the two dishes separated, then combine them and blend once more.
- Spoon hitter into the skillet.
- Cook for 20 minutes, or until brown with firm edges.
- Promptly turn the biscuits over utilizing a margarine blade. Leave them in the hot dish to keep the buildup from demolishing the surface.

3: Mixed Berry Chia Seed Pudding

Chia Seeds are a good source of fiber calcium, omega-3s, and iron. They likewise have limited quantities of phosphorous, manganese, potassium, and copper. I love their "crunchy" surface. They nearly help me to remember custard yet they're a lot better for you. Chia seeds can be eaten crudely or cooked.

I suggest eating them after they've either been drenched (like in a pudding recipe) or cooked because these seeds extend whenever they've been hydrated. Eating them dry can prompt them to extend in your throat which may give you a marginally abnormal inclination. One of the big advantages is the fiber content which will help give you a sensation of completion prompting better satiety.

Ingredients:

- 1/4 tsp vanilla embodiment
- 1 tsp. maple syrup
- 1 cup almond milk
- 1/4 cup white chia seeds (can use black)
- 1/2 cup characteristic Greek yogurt
- 1/4 tsp cinnamon
- 1/4 cup frozen OOB Organic blended berries

Method:

Into a little bowl, add chia seeds, yogurt, almond milk, honey, and vanilla concentrate

Mix well, as you don't need the chia to be staying together.

Cover, and leave in the ice chest short-term (or for 3+ hours).

Following two hours, give it another mix to guarantee it's all blending through.

Into a blender, add the chia combination (It should be thick at this point!) and the frozen berries.

Mix for 2-3 minutes, until your ideal consistency.

4: Gravy

This is a good fundamental recipe for the gravy, ideal for a Sunday broil. being an essential recipe, don't hesitate to trial and have a go at adding your ingredients, to your taste. for instance, this can be generally excellent with some milk or twofold cream mixed in, or without the wine added. for an alternate contort, add a squeeze or two of stew powder, for an additional kick! or on the other hand add some torn basil, coriander, or parsley.

Ingredients:

- 2 tbsp Flour
- 250ml Beef/Lamb broth
- 2 tbsp Beef/Lamb cooking juice
- Glug of Red Wine

Method:

- Put the cooking juice in a little container, and add the flour and a glug of red wine.
- Turn the pan on low - medium heat, and mix constantly. Don't let the sauce consume; this will destroy the flavor. you need a little steam falling off the outside of the fluid, yet not gurgling.
- Gradually add the stock, mixing meanwhile,until you accomplish the consistency you need.
- Keep on the heat until the gravy simply starts to bubble, yet not as much as a stew. Taste, andadd more stock, flour, or wine as liked.
- It is feasible to add salt and pepper at this stage. This tends not to be important, as a result of the flavoring in the cooking juice. If you do decide to add salt as well as pepper, do recollect what

the gravy is going to be poured over, and think about the general taste.

5: Eggplant Bacon

As a vegetable, eggplant doesn't have the best standing. However, this isn't because of the actual eggplant, this is a direct result of how it is habitually arranged. Breaded and singed, then layered with oily cheddar, eggplant unexpectedly turns into a caloric bad dream. The eggplant itself isn't high in calories, in any case.

It is comprised of 92% water and in this way contains just around 14 calories for every half cup all alone. It is likewise a good source of fiber, calcium, and potassium. So eggplant is an incredible decision to remember for your supper plate, and there are numerous sound and tasty approaches to set it up.

Eggplant sweethearts cheer—here's one all the more method to make the most of your number one purple-cleaned vegetable. Give this eggplant a shot crostino with a sprinkle of sliced tomatoes, feta, and tricks, or mix it into your #1 pasta with a sprinkle of good extra-virgin olive oil and a modest bunch of sliced basil.

Ingredients:

- Freshly ground black pepper
- 2 tbsp. extra-virgin olive oil
- 1 medium eggplant
- 2 tbsp. soy sauce

- 1/2 tsp. smoked paprika
- 1 tsp. maple syrup
- 1/2 tsp. Fluid Smoke

Method:

- Preheat broiler to 300°. Line 2 preparing sheets with material paper.
- Cut eggplant in quarters, longwise.
- Cut each quarter into long, flimsy strips.
- In a small bowl, whisk together soy sauce, olive oil, paprika, maple syrup, and fluid smoke.
- Spot eggplant cuts onto heating sheets and brushes the two sides with sauce. Season with pepper.
- Prepare until eggplant is cooked through and starting to get fresh, 45-50 minutes

6: Homemade Curry

Would you like to realize how to make simple curry that is loaded with healthy flavor and goodness that is modest and credible? Is it accurate to say that you are tired of paying great cash for exhausting and dull curries from your local cafés? Allow me to tell you the best way to make perhaps the best curry. All that curry can be an exquisite feast. A curry is ideal for supper or lunch. I have eaten numerous curries in my daily existence.

Unfortunately, I have eaten a lot of awful curries that have been made by individuals who should know better! A good curry shouldn't be costly. A good curry comprises fresh plans, spices, and flavors. The best thing about everything is that you will eat a homemade curry that is not difficult to make and is loaded up with sound spices and flavors.

Ingredients:

- curry leaf (10 leaves)
- ginger 2cm
- 300 grams of your #1 meat (marinate with a teaspoon of curry powder, sugar, teaspoon salt, and pepper for 2 hours before cooking)
- curry powder 300 grams
- 1 cup of coconut milk
- 1 teaspoon of pepper
- 50 grams dried chilies
- olive oil
- 2 garlic cloves
- 2 onions
- Indian Nan bread or supper bread rolls

Method:

- Heat a frying skillet with olive oil. Whenever it's warmed then add the garlic, curry leaf, onions, and ginger and mix until brilliant.
- Add your meat and mix for 2 minutes.
- In a 20-liter pot, add every one of the ingredients and cook for 2 hours under low heat.

- Mix the pot like clockwork to help theingredients blend and keep the lower part of thepot from consuming.
- Add the coconut milk toward the end and carry it to the bubble.
- To thicken the curry if it's not too much trouble, add cornflour in a little bowl and add a large part of some water.
- Blend this and afterward empty it into the pot and mix until the curry thickens.
- Topping with some fresh cream and coriander.

7: Bean Stew Seasoning

Potentially the least demanding because the essential ingredient is for some odd reason bean stew powder. Some you aware of everything might be thinking "Hello, bean stew powder is one of those pre-fabricated blends of a few flavors!" and you would be right however bean stew powder is fundamentally flavors and practically zero filler.

So back to the recipe, the stew powder will give you the bean stew flavor, then to add some profundity and smoky flavor we will add ground cumin, then you can add got dried out onions, garlic powder, and some other ingredient you think would round out the flavor profile that you need to make. There are a lot of plans for making "stew" preparing on the web.

Ingredients:

- 1 teaspoon cocoa powder
- 3 tablespoons bean stew powder
- 1 tablespoon ground cumin
- 1/2 teaspoon garlic powder
- 1/2 teaspoon onion powder
- 1/4 teaspoon cayenne pepper
- 1/2 teaspoon red pepper drops
- 1/4 teaspoon ground cinnamon
- 1 teaspoon paprika (use smoked paprika for a smokey contort)

Method:

- Combine all ingredients as one in a little bowl or container. Store in a little sealed shut holder.
- In the wake of cooking meat and vegetables for bean stew, mix in flavor blend and toast for 1-2 minutes before adding fluid ingredients to stew.

8: Date Syrup

The incredible thing about utilizing dates in your cooking is that it is flexible. You can use it in its strong state, as a thick puree, or in fluid-structure! You can use pretty much, contingent upon your preferences. Before utilizing dates in cooking plans consistently make sure that you pit them.

That implies eliminating the seed from within. It is not difficult to do and because the fruit is dry on the surface, there is no wreck included. Since the external skin of a date will in general solidify, particularly in cool environments, one valuable tip is to splash for a couple of moments in barely enough warm water. This isn't compulsory for all plans.

Date syrup is a well know sugar accessible today. Old cuneiform original copies from Mesopotamia notice the syrup, showing it as the essential sugar of that time. Thinking about the significant amount of date palms around there, it is likely this was alluding to honey from the date, or, date syrup.

Ingredient:

- 20 Medjool dates pitted
- 3 cups water

Method:

- Put the dates and water in a medium pot on medium-high heat to heat to the point of boiling.
- Then turn the heat down to medications low and let the blend stew.
- If you see froth showing up on the top, skim it off (the same thing you do when making soup broth, or jam).
- Utilizing a wooden spoon, blend sporadically and crush the dates with the rear of the spoon.
- After around 15 minutes of stewing, take it off the heat and let it cool.

9: Sirloin Steak

Sirloin steaks can give large cuts from 1.5 inches (37mm) to 2 inches (51mm) thick and are found to be for the most part the least expensive of the superior steaks. This is the reason this steak is generally well known among men and genuine grills. It is supposed that the name 'sirloin' was subsequently an English lord who was enamored with quality food and knight a piece of meat which he names 'sir midsection'. However, this is likely a miss-truth!

It is a unique sort of steak produced using hamburger meat that has been scaled from the back or back bit of the cow into its short flank. It includes the most sensitive and delectable meat a piece of the said creature, making it truly outstanding among the various steaks like t-bone, porterhouse, club steak, and such.

Ingredients:

- black pepper
- vegetable oil, or groundnut oil
- 2 sirloin steaks, estimating 3cm in thickness
- 1 handle of spread
- 1/4 pack of thyme
- flaky sea salt
- 3 garlic cloves, slammed yet unpeeled

Method:

- Before you start, reduce the steaks from the ice chest and let to come to room temperature (for at any rate 60 minutes)
- Preheat the stove to 180°C/gas mark 4
- Spot a substantially based skillet or iron dish over high heat and add a good scramble of oil.
- Season the steaks generously with flaky ocean salt
- When the oil is hot, add the steaks cautiously to the skillet and cook for 2 and a half minutes, or until wonderfully brilliant on the underside.
- Turn the steaks over and add a handle of spread, some thyme, and a couple of garlic cloves. Cookie the steak with the margarine and once brilliant on the underside, place on the stove for 2–3 minutes
- Reduce the steaks from the skillet and let to rest in a warm spot for 5 minutes before serving. Season and serve

10: Cereal Banana Waffle

A waffle is a kind of cake like a hotcake. They are for the most part prepared between two hot plates. Cooking the two sides simultaneously. This gives them an inside and out crunchy outside and a uniform tone. They are the most broadly had breakfast food on the planet. The fan top pick anyway is the Oatmeal Banana Waffle. It very well might be a direct result of its abundant resources that trap products of the soil so you get a ton in one chomp.

Ingredients:

- 2 cups water
- 2 cups oats
- 1/2 banana
- 2 tablespoons olive oil
- 2 tablespoons powdered milk
- 1/2 teaspoon salt

Method:

- Turn waffle iron on high
- Put ingredients in the blender and mix on high until the substance are smooth
- Allow the blend to sit for a couple of moments to thicken
- Shower the waffle iron with a non-poisonous non-stick splash
- Pour the blend on to the waffle iron
- Cook for around 10 minutes
- Rehash until you are out of the player

11: North Staffordshire Oatcakes

North Staffordshire oatcakes are a local delicacy in the North Staffordshire space of England, thus might be referred to non-local people as a North Staffordshire oatcake or Potteries oatcake. These utilize flour and yeast, though different oatcakes don't.

When pre-cooked, they are a type of inexpensive food, and catering outlets in the space generally offer oatcakes with fillings like cheddar, bacon, wiener, and egg. They can be re-warmed by fricasseeing in margarine, or by flame broiling. What's more, pikelets are frequently served close by oatcakes also.

Ingredients:

- 8oz fine oats
- 1 teaspoon salt
- 8oz whole-wheat or plain flour
- 1/2oz fresh yeast
- 1 teaspoon sugar
- 1/2 pints' warm milk and water, blended cream

Method:

- Add the salt to the flour and oats.
- Break up the yeast with somewhat warm fluid and add the sugar. Let the blend get foamy.
- Blend the dry ingredients with the yeast fluid to make a hitter.
- Cover the hitter with a spotless material and leave it in a warm spot for 60 minutes.
- Prepare the oatcake on an all-around lubed iron. Put sufficient player onto the frying pan to create an oatcake around 8-9 creeps in breadth. The surface will be canvassed in openings as it cooks.
- Turn the oatcake following 2 - 3 minutes when the upper side seems dry and the under is brilliant brown, and cook for another 2 - 3 minutes.

12: Cereal Raisin Cookies

The word 'oats raisin cookies' carries water to the mouth and fills the nostrils with its warm smell. Allow us to examine the recipe of oats raisin cookies, how grandmother used to make, with a slight variation. Since many keep away from eggs but then many are sensitive to drain items, we will get ready vegetarian cereal raisin cookies.

The flavor challenges depiction and the fragrance of them heating will transform even the most current of kitchen spaces into a Donna Reed-time cooking retail outlet. Don't be amazed if you end up battling the staggering desire to tie on a gingham cover while the blending and preparing measure happens.

Ingredients:

- 1/3 c water or milk
- 1/2 tsp vanilla
- 1/4 c brown sugar - immovably stuffed
- 3/4 c spread, fruit purée, a balance of margarine and vegetable oil, or shortening
- 1 egg
- 3c oats, moved (crude) - fast/antiquated
- 1/2 tsp heating pop
- 1 c flour - universally handy
- 1/2 tsp salt
- 1c raisins
- 3/4 c pecans - sliced
- 1/4 tsp cinnamon

Method:

- Heat broiler to 350°F.
- Delicately oil cookie sheet with oil.
- Consolidate margarine, fruit purée, spread/vegetable oil blend, or shortening, brown sugar, milk, egg, and vanilla; beat with the blender on fast to mix well.

- Consolidate oats, flour, heating pop, salt, and cinnamon; add to the shortening combination and join until just mixed.
- Mix in raisins and nuts.
- Drop by adjusted tablespoonful onto lubed cookie sheet, 2 inches separated.
- Prepare for 10-13 min., or until gently cooked.

13: Chai Tea Latte

There is certainly something exceptional about a Chai Tea Latte. For individuals who are stuck in a rut and who need to adhere to moment espresso or normal tea that might be a genuine disgrace because without taking a stab at something fresh, you don't have the foggiest idea of what you are absent. It is in every case great to try fresh things throughout everyday life.

It is extraordinary being somewhat gutsy with your food and beverages, although I would resist the urge to stress about the hard beverages. Chai tea latte is a quieting drink arranged without any preparation using a chai combination. Furthermore, we have arranged a few stages to make a reviving beverage of chai tea latte.

Ingredients:

- 2 black tea sacks (optional; I like to use Darjeeling)
- 2 cups almond milk (or milk of decision)
- 3/4 teaspoon ground cinnamon, or to taste
- 1/4 teaspoon ground ginger
- 3 tablespoons maple syrup (or sugar of decision)
- 1/8 teaspoon ground cloves

Method:

- In the case of utilizing tea, remember that this beverage will have caffeine.
- Heat the almond milk in a pot over medium-high heat, until it starts to rise around the edges of the skillet.
- Mood killer the heat, and add the 2 tea packs to the pot of hot milk.
- Hang tight 3 to 5 minutes for the tea to steep, then reduce the packs and proceed with the following stage.
- In case you're skirting the tea, add the plain almond milk to a sauce skillet.
- Since the milk is in the pot (regardless of whether it's been blended as tea, or not) include the cinnamon, cloves, ginger, and maple syrup.
- Race to join, mixing over medium heat, until the blend is steaming hot.
- Change any flavoring as you would prefer and serve right away.
- Extras can be store in a water/airproof compartment for as long as 4 days in the refrigerator.
- You can serve them chilled over ice, or warm on the oven once more.

Chapter: 2 Lunch

14: Simply Granola Bars

Everyone likes granola bars yet did you realize that they are really basic and modest to make at home? When you make homemade granola bars you can tweak the flavor and surface to suit your specific preferences and you can make them as nutritious or wanton as you can imagine.

The recipe is essential and just requires a couple of moments of hands-on readiness followed by a speedy outing through the stove. Toward the end, you have a tremendous plate of heavenly tidbits that will save pleasantly in a covered holder for at any rate seven days. By exploring different avenues regarding ingredients you can make fresh flavors and surfaces.

Ingredients:

- 3 eggs
- 1/3 cup brown sugar (discard if granola is extremely sweet)
- 3/4 cup softened spread or margarine
- 1 teaspoon vanilla
- 1/2 teaspoon salt
- 4 cups granola cereal

Method:

- Preheat the broiler to 400 degrees. In a blending bowl, combine as one softened margarine and sugar.

- Add vanilla, salt, and eggs.
- Beat until smooth.
- Mix in granola and press into a lubed 9x13 heating dish.
- Heat in the broiler for 15 to 20 minutes or until all-around set.
- Cool and cut into bars.
- These are flat-out genuine cookies and particularly pleasant if you have made a strawberry or peach jam throughout the mid-year.
- In this after recipe, carob powder is used.
- Carob is regularly called 'the chocolate substitute." It makes prepared products dull and damp.
- It is produced using the case of the carob tree, also called St. John's bread.

It is low in fat, high in protein and minerals.

15: Chocolate Brownie

Such a Chocolatey chocolate brownie that must be accomplished by good natural cocoa and chocolate. Such a Chocolatey chocolate brownie that increases in flavor if you leave them in a tin for a little while. This recipe also bends over as a hot pudding for a cold winter's day, it is brilliant hot with frozen yogurt over it, however, use an espresso or vanilla frozen yogurt as a rich chocolate one takes away from the kind of the brownie.

Ingredients:

- 250g spread
- 300g caster sugar
- 3 large natural eggs in addition to an extra egg yolk
- 250g chocolate
- 60g flour
- ½ tsp preparing powder
- 60g great quality natural cocoa powder

Method:

- Oil the preparing plate with margarine.
- Put the sugar and spread it into the bowl of a food blender and cream them together for a few minutes until they are pale and feathery.
- Put a bowl over a dish of boiling water, yet make sure that the lower part of the bowl doesn't contact the water, or the chocolate will go grainy when it dissolves.
- Keep 50g to the side and break the rest into little parts and leave it in the bowl over the water.
- Leave it for five minutes and mix, when it has liquefied reduce it from the heat.
- Break the excess 50g into pieces the size of big full raisins.
- Beat the eggs gently in a little bowl.
- Strainer together the flour, cocoa, and heating powder to reduce the irregularities and make it

light and vaporous, add a spot of rock salt to escalate the kind of chocolate.

- Add the eggs to the creamed spread and sugar a little at a time, it will sour if you add everything simultaneously.
- When the egg has all been fusing, overlap in the liquefied chocolate and the chopped chocolate.
- Delicately overlap in the flour and cocoa, do this gradually, and don't exhaust, as you should be certain not to take the air out of the flour blend.
- Fill the readied dish or heating tin and shake on the worktop, to level the top marginally.
- Heat for around thirty minutes, the chocolate brownies are prepared when the edge is pulling somewhat away from the dish, however, the middle looks delicate and squiggly.
- If you don't know embed a metal stick in the middle and it should arise marginally wet, however not with crude combination adhering to it.
- Brownies proceed to cook and set in the tin when cooling so make sure that it isn't overcooked.
- If it isn't exactly prepared, return it to the stove yet check each a few minutes.

16: Taco Seasoning

Tacos are scrumptious and are made to go with lunch and supper, or similarly as a side dish if you like to. Then you can add tomato, onion, sharp cream, fresh guacamole and you can finish off it with anything you like. Imagine how delectable these tacos will be and they will be caused with all the stuff you to feel are astounding together.

Ingredients:

- 5 teaspoons paprika
- 6 teaspoons bean stew powder
- 4 1/2 teaspoons cumin
- 3 teaspoons onion powder
- 2 1/2 teaspoons garlic powder
- 1/4 teaspoon cayenne pepper

Method:

- Join all ingredients together, and blend well. This should be store in a water/airproof compartment for as long as a half year.
- You can change this recipe, here and there I like to add some oregano to my blend.
- Smoked chipotle peppers and ancho pepper are likewise pleasant increments, as they will make heavenly flavors.
- Perhaps the best thing about making your zest mix is that you will change and alter the recipe for your preferences.
- If you like zesty food, you can add more cayenne pepper. If you don't care for it so fiery, you can avoid the cayenne pepper about the recipe.

- To use this flavoring blend, basically use 3 tablespoons and some water whenever you have sautéed one pound of ground hamburger.
- Essentially add the flavoring blend, and water, and let the water decrease by 1/2 and you have a few tacos that have been prepared impeccably, and you did it all yourself without purchasing a business blend.

17: Mama yo (Vegan Mayonnaise)

Delightful vegetarian mayo, made with just 4 ingredients and in only 2 minutes! This vegetarian mayonnaise is so scrumptious, velvety, rich, and without cholesterol. Making vegetarian mayo is so natural, it just requires 4 ingredients, only 2 minutes, and a blender, there's nothing more to it.

A submersion blender is the most ideal decision; however, a normal blender will do. This vegetarian mayonnaise is made without milk or eggs. It tastes incredible as a plunge with veggies or on bread. Store in a shut compartment in the cooler for as long as about fourteen days.

Ingredients:

- 1/2 tsp salt
- 1/2 cup unsweetened soy milk (125 ml)
- 1 cup oil (250 ml)
- 2 tsp apple juice vinegar

Method:

- Make sure the oil is at a similar temperature as the milk. You can use cold oil and cold milk, however, I discovered room temperature milk and oil to be the simplest to work with.
- In case you're utilizing an inundation blender, join every one of the ingredients in the blender cup, place the submersion blender in, so way it sits solidly on the lower part of the cup, and heartbeat until the mayo emulsifies.
- When the greater part of the veggie lover mayo has emulsified, you can move the blender here and there to consolidate any oil that is perched on the top.
- In case you're utilizing a standard blender, place every one of the ingredients in the blender, except the oil, and mix for around 5 seconds.
- Then add the oil progressively while the blender is going at a sluggish speed until it thickens, then you can divert it steadily from low to high and let it go until all around blended.
- Try the mayo and add more salt if necessary. If it's excessively thick, add more milk, and if it's too watery add more oil.
- Heartbeat again until the mayo has the ideal consistency.
- Use it promptly or save it in the refrigerator for a couple of hours until it's cold. Keep extras in a water/airproof compartment or a container in the refrigerator for around 4-7 days.

18: Taco Stuffed Peppers

This speedy and simple supper recipe makes certain to satisfy the whole family! Peppers loaded up with the best taco meat, finished off with cheddar, and the very best taco ingredients. In case you're longing for tacos however not all the carbs, you'll love these eased-up stuffed peppers.

The peppers are burrowed out and simmered in the stove, then loaded down with ground hamburger, black beans, brown rice, corn, and salsa. It's beginning and end you love about tacos, all in a consumable vegetable bowl. You can generally trade ground meat for chicken or turkey, or stick to rice and keep this recipe vegan.

Ingredients:

- extra-virgin olive oil
- 1 clove garlic, crushed
- 1/2 Onion, sliced (around 1 cup)
- 1 lb. ground hamburger
- Freshly ground black pepper
- adequate salt
- 2 tbsp. Sliced cilantro
- 1/2 tsp. ground cumin
- 1 tsp. bean stew powder
- 1/2 tsp. smoked paprika
- 1 c. smashed Cheddar
- 3 ringer peppers, split (seeds reduced)
- 1 c. Smashed Monterey Jack

- Hot sauce, for serving
- 1 c. Smashed lettuce
- Pico de gallo, for serving
- Lime wedges, for serving

Method:

- Preheat the broiler to 375° and splash a big heating dish with a cooking shower.
- In a big skillet over medium heat, heat around 1 tablespoon olive oil.
- Add onion and cook until the onion is delicate around 5 minutes.
- Mix in garlic. Cook it until fragrant
- Add ground meat and cook until not, at this point pink, around 5 minutes. Channel fat.
- Add ground cumin, bean stew powder, and paprika to hamburger blend, then season with salt and pepper.
- Sprinkle ringer peppers with olive oil and season with salt and pepper.
- Spot the peppers, cut side up, in the heating dish, and spoon meat combination into each pepper.
- Top with cheddar and prepare until the cheddar is liquefied and the peppers are fresh delicate, around 20 minutes.
- Top each pepper with lettuce and present with pico de gallo, hot sauce, and lime wedges.

19: Chicken Tagine with Prunes and Almonds

Food in Morocco assumes a significant part in customary life. From weddings to sanctifications to circumcisions, it is the premise of get-togethers and festivities. From couscous to tagines and pastilles, the fragile flavors are a mix of tastes of numerous human advancements. A conventional Moroccan dish is a tagine, a stew of vegetables with poultry or meat and dried fruit.

The fruit is added towards the finish to give general pleasantness to the dish. The vegetables are set around the meat, which is set in the focal point of the pot along with the fruit. The tagine is then covered and cooked gradually over a charcoal oven

Ingredient:

- 1 chicken, cut up into 6 pieces
- 170 g (6 oz) dried prunes, chopped fine
- 60 g (2 oz) whole, whitened almonds
- 1 large white onion, finely sliced 2 cloves of garlic, squashed
- ½ teaspoon powdered ginger
- 1 teaspoon powdered cinnamon
- ½ teaspoon turmeric
- 1 teaspoon ground cumin
- 2 tablespoons vegetable oil
- salt and freshly ground black pepper to taste

Method:

- The following, set up the chicken marinade.
- Wash the chicken in salted water and channel.
- Blend squashed garlic in with 1 tbsp. salt to make glue.
- Rub into the chicken and afterward flush under running water until the chicken no longer scents of garlic.
- Channel and store.
- Rub the chicken pieces with cumin, salt, and pepper and let represent 60 minutes.
- Cover the prunes with cold water, add the cinnamon and bring to the bubble.
- Cover and stew for 30 minutes or more - until the prunes are delicate.
- Spot the chicken pieces in a 5-quart profound meal over medium heat and add the chopped onion, ginger, turmeric, salt, pepper, and almonds.
- When the almonds are brown, reduce with a punctured spoon and
- channel on kitchen paper.
- When the chicken is seared, cover with water just so the chicken pieces are covered and bring to the bubble.
- Reduce heat and stew, covered, for 30 minutes.
- Following 30 minutes, add the prunes and a part of the prune water to the goulash and keep cooking until the chicken and prunes are extremely delicate.

- Sprinkle with the almonds and serve on the double.

20: Lemon Iced Tea

Tea has no calories, however, it has heaps of cancer prevention agents in fundamental basic Fresh tea, and even it will assist you with losing weight. To get the nutritious employments of it you need to try it at home as per your taste. Here is a healthy summer seasoned tea plan and enhanced frosted tea syrups and you can likewise make unsweetened tea recipes.

Making tea is peaceful and simple; you can drink it light or healthy, drink it without sugar or with sugar. Whenever you have the basics, you can begin getting innovative - simply follow the simple strides beneath. You can use seasoned frosted tea sacks.

Ingredients:

- 1 ¼ cups sugar
- 2 big lemons
- 2 cups fresh mint leaves, in addition to additional for decorating
- ½ cup fresh lemon juice
- 6 black tea packs

Method:

- Utilizing a vegetable peeler, reduce dazzling yellow strip from lemons.
- Join lemon strip and sugar in a medium pan with 1/2 cup water and heat to the point of boiling, blending to break up sugar.
- Lower heat and stew for 2 minutes.
- Reduce from heat and mix in mint.
- Cool to room temperature; strain.
- Steep the tea packs in 4 cups of bubbling water, covered, for 5 minutes.
- Then reduce tea packs.
- Mix in syrup, 4 cups cold water, lemon squeeze, and ice healthy shapes.
- Serve in tall glasses loaded up with ice and a couple of mint leaves.

21: Ratatouille

Comprised of a wide range of vegetables, ratatouille is generally tantamount to a vegetable stew. An adaptable dish by its own doing: it tends to be served hot, cold, or even tepid. Consider it an hors d'oeuvre, consider it your principal course, anything you desire to call it, it's an exemplary French dish, to be specific from the Provencal district.

Some serve it with fundamentals, others on a bed of rice. Ratatouille bears no weight of limitations. Furthermore, for all you extra darlings, many fight that ratatouille tastes better the day after it is cooked. Chocolate and Zucchini even consider it an "ideal make-ahead dish." So give it a shot.

Ingredients:

- 1/4 cup olive oil, in addition, to add on a case by case basis
- 1 little eggplant, sliced
- Legitimate salt and freshly ground black pepper
- 1 zucchini, chopped
- 3 little tomatoes, chopped
- 1 pepper (red, green, or yellow), sliced
- 1 onion, sliced
- 3 cloves garlic, squeezed
- 3 or 4 leaves fresh basil, sliced
- 2 teaspoons sliced fresh thyme
- Sprinkle red wine vinegar

Method:

- Heat 2 tablespoons of oil in a large skillet or Dutch broiler.

- Cook the vegetables each in turn (independently) for 5 to 7 minutes, adding somewhat more oil on a case by case basis and preparing with salt, in the accompanying request: onion, zucchini, eggplant, pepper, and tomatoes.
- Consolidate the whole of the cooked vegetables together in the skillet, thyme, add the garlic, and basil and let stew delicately for 20 minutes.
- Add a sprinkle of red wine vinegar, season with salt and pepper, and afterward turn off the heat.
- Serve hot, warm, or cold.

22: Avocado Egg Cups

Although avocados start from Mexico and Central America they were purchased to Spain by the conquistadors and have adjusted well to the Mediterranean environment and develop here in bounty. They are a surprising and valuable fruit since they don't as expect mature until picked so can be left on the tree and be gathered throughout the whole year.

Already they have been found to have umpteen medical advantages and as they are incorporated routinely in the Mediterranean diet they give further weight to the well-being giving advantages of this diet.

Ingredients:

- 6 big whole egg
- 3 Avocado
- 6 cut Uncured Turkey Bacon

Method:

- Slice the main avocado down the middle and scoop out the seed. Scoop out a part of the avocado to make space for the eggs.
- Rehash these means for the excess two avocados.
- Preheat the broiler to 425 degrees Fahrenheit.
- Spot the avocado parts on a biscuit tin and break 1 egg in every avocado.
- Heat for 14 to 16 minutes, or until the eggs are cooked as you would prefer.
- Top with cooked, uncured turkey bacon - one strip for every avocado half.

23: Scaled Down Frittatas

There is by all accounts a touch of conversation about what a frittata (articulated 'free-TAH-tah) truly is. Is it a kind of quiche, or is it an omelet? To give the initial two definitions, a quiche regularly is an egg dish made with cream prepared in an outside layer, practically like a pie. A quiche can have an assortment of ingredients added into it to make various styles and tastes.

An omelet, on the other hand, is just beaten eggs cooked with spread or oil in a griddle with the hardened egg collapsed around different ingredients. Average omelet ingredients incorporate cheddar, onions, bacon, mushrooms, different vegetables, ham, or different meats.

Frittatas can contain quite a few unique ingredients. Fresh vegetables, mushrooms, cheeses, meat, potatoes, various spices, or any mix thereof are normal. Extra vegetables or cooked meat are likewise incredible in frittatas. Spices, fresh or dried, can likewise add a great deal of flavor to a frittata, or you could use your number one hot pepper sauce to zest it up too.

Ingredients:

- 3/4 cup salsa
- 1-1/2 cups frozen smashed hash brown potatoes, defrosted
- 1 Italian turkey hotdog connect (around 4 ounces), packaging reduced
- 1/2 cup chopped onion
- 1 teaspoon canola oil
- 1/3 cup water
- 1 garlic clove, crushed
- 1/2 teaspoon salt
- 1/2 to 1 teaspoon dried oregano
- 1/4 teaspoon pepper
- 3 large eggs
- 1/2 teaspoon dried thyme
- 2 big egg whites

- 2 tablespoons universally handy flour
- 1 cup buttermilk
- 1/4 cup smashed Parmesan cheddar

Method:

- In a nonstick skillet, cook frankfurter over medium heat until not, at this point pink.
- Reduce with an opened spoon to paper towels. Dispose of drippings.
- In a similar skillet, sauté potatoes, onion, and garlic in oil until potatoes are brilliant brown, around 5 minutes.
- Add water, flavors and hotdog; cook and mix over medium heat until the water has vanished, around 1 moment.
- In a bowl, consolidate the eggs, egg whites, buttermilk, flour, and Parmesan cheddar.
- Mix in hotdog combination. Fill biscuit cups covered with cooking splash three-fourths full.
- Prepare at 350° for 20-25 minutes or until a blade confesses all.
- Thoroughly run a blade around the edge of cups to extricate frittatas.
- Present with salsa.

Chapter: 3 Dinner

24: Pasta and Summer Vegetables Recipe

If you read my recipe for Tomato Salad, you realize that I love the late spring. I trust you do likewise. Throughout the late spring, everything is simply blasting around you. Vegetables are at their pinnacle of readiness and flavor. Everything is simply so acceptable. You never consider wintertime and the lower evaluation of vegetables that are accessible. If you have a nursery, you can develop all that is in this dish. Hence, it will be greatly improved.

Ingredients:

- 1 Medium Zucchini
- 3 Large, Blood Red Native Tomatoes
- 1 Medium Onion. Red, Yellow or White
- 1 Yellow Squash
- Garlic Cloves
- 7 Fresh Basil Leafs, Torn
- Olive oil, salt, and pepper
- Hard Italian bread
- ½ pounds of dry pasta
- Ground Parmesan cheddar

Method:

- Carry a Large Pot of water to the bubble. Salt the water generously and cook the pasta until Al Dente. Somewhat hard.

- While trusting that the word will bubble and keeping in mind that the pasta is cooking, do stages 2-9
- Coarsely Chop the Tomato, store
- Slice the zucchini down the middle the long way and afterward into equal parts longwise once more. Coarsely cleave, store
- Do likewise for the Yellow Squash, store
- Coarsely dice the onion, store
- Coarsely slash the garlic, store
- In a griddle on medium/high, sauté the onion and garlic until marginally delicate.
- Spot the Zucchini and Yellow Squash in with the onion and garlic. Sauté until marginally relaxed
- Yet, the tomatoes in the griddle and sauté until mollified marginally
- Spot the pasta in the griddle alongside 1-2 Ladle's of pasta water
- Cook everything on Medium/High heat until the vegetables are marginally more relaxed. 3-5 minutes
- Mood killer them and toss in the basil and throw.

25: Green Beans and Almonds

Fresh green beans should be fresh and break effectively when they are bowed. If the green bean creases over effectively it isn't just about as fresh as it should be. It can in any case be used however the freshness of the bean is no more. There isn't anything more delectable than great fresh green bean plans and I will give you a part of my top picks.

Before I get into the plans I might want to reveal to you how you can freeze fresh green beans. Spot the beans in a sifter and whiten with extremely boiling water. Quickly place the beans in a plastic cooler pack and spot them in your cooler on the rack where you would put all moment freeze food sources.

Ingredients:

- 1/2 stick of spread
- 2 lbs. of fresh green beans
- 1 cup of toasted almonds less if you don't care for a lot of almonds
- Salt and pepper to taste

Method:

- Wash and reduce the string from the green beans and snap off the finishes.
- Bubble or steam the green beans until cooked yet fresh
- In a skillet dissolve the margarine and add the cooked green beans
- Blend well and add the almonds and salt and pepper.
- Combine the whole of the ingredients as one well and on a low fire let the combination
- Cook until done however the beans are as yet fresh.

26: Chicken Pork Adobo

Being perhaps the most loved food variety of Filipinos, the adobo has a few varieties. The chicken pork adobo is a recipe that is consistently present in the weekly menus of families since it is a mix of two of the most cherished meats for the Pinoy sense of taste.

It also works to the upside of mothers who get befuddled between pork adobo and chicken adobo because there is no more need to settle on a decision between the two. For my situation, my better half loves pork adobo while my child consistently demands chicken adobo. To fulfill them both, I generally wind up cooking chicken pork adobo as well.

Ingredients:

- 3 tablespoons salt
- 1/4 pounds' pork flank broil (boneless and cut into 2-inch pieces)
- 1/4 pounds' chicken bosoms (boneless, skinless, and cut into 2-inch pieces)
- 2 cloves garlic (crushed)
- 2 inlet leaves (torn)
- 2 tablespoons squashed garlic
- 1 tablespoon black peppercorns (coarsely ground)
- 1 tablespoon vegetable oil
- 1 cup white vinegar
- 1/4 cup soy sauce (optional)

Method:

- Use salt and pepper to prepare the chicken and pork meat.
- Then put all the meat in a broth pot. Add the torn cove leaf and squashed garlic.
- Coat with white vinegar and soy sauce.
- Cover the pot and spot it in the cooler for at any rate 8 hours or overnight to marinate.
- Cook under medium-high heat and heat to the point of boiling.
- Then decrease heat and stew until meat is delicate when tried with a fork, as a rule, takes around 1 ½ hour.
- To prevent drying out, add a little measure of water whenever required.
- Reduce the meat from the cooking fluid.
- Spot the fluid back to the broth pot and let stew.
- Over medium-high heat, cook the meat in vegetable oil while mixing.
- Continue cooking until every one of the sides of the meat becomes brown.
- Just now after cooking, add the leftover crushed garlic.
- Add every one of the meats to the stewing fluid and cook until the sauce is marginally thickened.
- Serve hot with plain white rice.

27: Best Veggie Broth

Vegetable broth is an economical and healthy approach to add flavor to a wide range of suppers. Save extra vegetables, scraps, and spices in a big cooler sack until you have enough to make the stock. Examination with various vegetable mixes to track down the best flavor. Freeze broth in more modest segments for simple and fast access. Broth can be frozen in an ice 3D shape plate and afterward moved to cooler packs.

Ingredients:

- 8 cups water
- 1 inlet leaf
- 2 medium onions, cut into wedges
- 2 tablespoons olive oil
- 2 celery ribs, cut into 1-inch pieces
- 3 medium leeks, white and light green parts just, cleaned and cut into 1-inch pieces
- 1 whole garlic bulb, isolated into cloves, and stripped
- 1/2 pound fresh mushrooms, quartered
- 1 cup pressed fresh parsley branches
- 1 teaspoon salt
- 3 medium carrots, cut into 1-inch pieces
- 4 branches fresh thyme
- 1/2 teaspoon whole peppercorns

Method:

- Heat oil in a stockpot over medium heat until hot.
- Add celery, onions, and garlic.
- Cook and mix for 5 minutes or until delicate.

- Add leeks and carrots; cook and mix for 5 minutes.
- Add water, parsley, mushrooms, salt, peppercorns thyme, and cove leaf; heat to the point of boiling.
- Lessen heat; stew, revealed, 60 minutes.
- Reduce from heat.
- Strain through a cheesecloth-lined colander; dispose of vegetables.
- In the case of utilizing quickly, skim fat. Or on the other hand, refrigerate for 8 hours or overnight; reduce fat from the surface.
- Broth can be concealed and refrigerated for 3 days or frozen as long as a half year.

28: Creole

Tomatoes and shrimp concocted with garlic and onions - this Gulf Coast custom will make them long for the narrows. This recipe can either be a fundamental dish or a side dish. You can make it as hot as you need, simply add more stew powder and hot sauce. Serve over hot rice. This Creole dish is cooked with tomatoes, onions, peppers, and celery. Change the zest to your inclination, yet don't be frightened of a little heat.

To the plan of the best jambalaya recipe, here is a customary Creole Jambalaya recipe that will undoubtedly stimulate the taste buds.

Ingredients:

- About 142grams of chicken cut them into about 2.5cmsq. 3D shapes
- 2 and ½ cups of rice
- About 85grams of pork ribs, cut the same size as the chicken. Smoked pork doesn't work!
- About 170grams of Andouille hotdog suggested yet replacements will do if inaccessible in the nearby market
- About 142grams of ham healthy shapes
- About 343grams of crude shelled shrimps
- 1 and ½ cups of finely sliced onions
- A 0.35l of hand squashed tomatoes, an unquestionable requirement!
- 1/2 cup of finely sliced red chime pepper
- 1 cup of finely sliced celery
- 1 cup of finely sliced green chime pepper
- 6 cloves of squashed or squeezed garlic
- Clam or vegetable juice, depending on the situation - No water!
- 2 cups of chicken broth
- ½ tablespoon every one of white, red, and black peppers
- ¼ teaspoon of finger-squashed saffron
- 1 tablespoon of pale dry sherry, whenever wanted
- ¼ teaspoon of monosodium glutamate
- ¼ teaspoon of thyme
- 3 tablespoon of Spanish olive oil, an absolute necessity
- 1 and ½ teaspoons of Hungarian HOT paprika

- 1 little cove leave

Method:

- Heat the olive oil in the Cast Iron Pot or a Dutch stove
- Add the peppers, onion, garlic, and celery and mix, cook on high flares until ingredients are clear
- Add the chicken and pork and continue to mix until they become white
- Add the Ham and wiener and mix for about 3minutes
- Add the tomatoes and mix for 5minutes
- Lower the heat to medium and add the chicken broth and mix
- With the same heat, add a wide range of various flavors aside from the sherry in any request and mix.
- Let to cook for about 20minutes.
- Add the rice
- Cover the pot
- Cook for about 30minutes
- Add the shrimp and the sherry
- If necessary or if the rice isn't all around cooked, add the Vegetable or Clam squeeze and mix it all. Let to cook for another 5 to 10minutes
- Mood killer the heat and let it stew and serve

29: The Ultimate Acai Berry

The ubiquity of the Acai Berry Smoothie is obvious; indeed, you can see it advanced anyplace, from chocolates, juices, lunchrooms, and even wellbeing drinks. You would now be able to make your own Acai smoothie. It very well may be effortlessly arranged and it is ideal for your wellbeing.

If you are experiencing difficulty getting your children, or even yourself, to eat or drink whatever's healthy for them, why not let them try this. You can get every one of the advantages of the berry from this beverage and it is the ideal method to get going your day and give you that additional charge you need.

The ingredients are not definite, yet just estimated since you need to think about your taste when making this. Aside from that, as long as you put in the berries, then you can choose the amount of what you will add. This recipe serves around two individuals, so you can make so a lot or as little as you need.

Ingredients:

- Void two Acai cases into it or a teaspoon of acai powder.
- 6-7 strawberries
- 1/2 cup blueberries
- 2 scoops of non-fat vanilla frozen yogurt

Method:

- Put the strawberries and the blueberries in the blender.
- Mix them until they are smooth, except if you need to have some chunkier pieces.
- Add the two scoops of vanilla frozen yogurt into the blender, and mix away alongside the berries.
- Open two containers of the Acai and empty the substance into the blender under a low setting.
- This will help with guaranteeing an intensive blend.
- And afterward, the whole of that is left is a major good glass of Acai smoothie only for you.

30: Marinara Sauce Recipe

Here is an extraordinary recipe for marinara sauce utilizing canned tomatoes. This marinara sauce is delectable over your #1 pasta, on top of pizza, and over mussels and shrimp. The excellence of this sauce is that it tends to be used with various plans, so it's an extraordinary beginning stage in Italian Cooking and it is not difficult to make.

You can use either fresh or canned plum tomatoes for this recipe, anyway utilizing fresh tomatoes requires additional time and planning, so I like to use canned. If you do anticipate utilizing fresh tomatoes, make certain the tomatoes are ready and in season.

For the canned tomatoes, I lean toward Rienzi brand tomatoes. I have tried various brands of canned tomatoes and Rienzi has the best flavor among the grocery store brands, as I would see it.

Ingredients:

- 1/4 cup extra virgin olive oil
- 1 35-ounce jar of whole plum tomatoes with fluid
- 4 garlic cloves, stripped and sliced (More or less relying upon the amount you like garlic)
- Salt to taste
- 10 - 12 fresh basil leaves, torn
- Squashed red pepper to taste
- 1/2 teaspoon of dried oregano

Method:

- Open your container of tomatoes and squash them by hand into a bowl and store.
- Medium heat the olive oil in a big pan.
- Add your garlic to the oil and cook until delicate and daintily sautéed.
- Make sure to watch the garlic to ignite sure it doesn't.
- Cautiously add the tomatoes alongside their fluid into the dish with garlic and oil.
- Use alarm while adding the tomatoes to the hot oil. The oil can splatter.
- Add the oregano.
- Mix the blend and heat to the point of boiling.
- Season with a touch of salt and red or black pepper.

- Lower the heat so the sauce is reduced to a stew.
- Separate the tomatoes as it cooks with a spoon until your sauce is thick.
- You need the sauce to stew until thickened, around 20 - 25 minutes.
- Add your fresh basil a couple of moments before the sauce is finished.
- Taste the sauce
- Add more salt or pepper if necessary.
- Serve over your favorite pasta.

31: Pesto Sauce Recipe

This is another extremely simple and delightful recipe that can be served over your number one pasta, grilled chicken, mussels, or as an ingredient for pizza. For a good minor departure from this recipe, have a go at adding sundried tomatoes to the pesto combination before mixing for a delectable tomato pesto sauce.

This recipe is a guide for you. Not every person has similar inclinations. Some don't care for a lot of garlic or olive oil flavor for instance, so it is suggested that you try until you track down the correct recipe.

Ingredients:

- 3/4 cup sliced pecans or pine nuts (the nuts can be daintily toasted in a dry skillet before mixing for added flavor)
- 4 cups fresh basil leaves
- 2 cloves garlic, stripped and chopped (pretty much relying upon your taste)
- 1/2 cup of extra virgin olive oil
- 1/2 cup of ground Parmesan cheddar
- salt and pepper to taste

Method:

- Add all ingredients to blender (except olive oil.)
- Add a little oil at once until sauce arrives at the wanted consistency.

Prepared to serve in your number one dish.

32: Simple Pasta with Garlic, Oil, and Fresh Herbs

This is another fast and simple Italian recipe with a couple of ingredients. Significantly, you don't consume the garlic with this recipe else it will turn out to be harsh.

Ingredients:

- 1 pound of spaghetti
- 1/2 cup held pasta water
- 3 - 4 garlic cloves sliced

- 1/4 Cup of Chopped Italian Flat Leaf Parsley
- 6 tablespoons of extra virgin olive oil
- 1/4 cup of sliced fresh basil leaves
- A spot of red pepper pieces
- Salt to taste

Method:

- In a large pot, achieve 6 quarts of salted water to a moving bubble.
- Add the pasta and cook for around 6 - 8 minutes or until still somewhat firm.
- Channel however make sure you save around 1/2 cup of pasta water.
- Heat 4 tablespoons of olive oil (while the pasta is cooking) over medium heat in a large skillet.
- Add the garlic and sauté until light brown in shading.
- Make sure to give close consideration to the garlic to ignite sure it doesn't.
- Reduce from heat.
- Mix in fresh spices, red pepper drops, and few tablespoons of the saved pasta water.
- Blend until joined.
- Move the depleted pasta to a big serving bowl and blend in the excess olive oil and pasta water.
- Add the garlic and spice combination into the pasta and blend well.
- Taste and add salt and red pepper whenever wanted.

- Serve right away. Top with ground cheddar whenever wanted.

33: Sicilian Succo

Ground hamburger and ground pork meatballs are seared in olive oil and served over a rich pureed tomato in this conventional Sicilian recipe. You can substitute zucchini for the meatballs for a veggie lover variant.

Ingredients:

- 1 tsp garlic powder
- 3 (29-oz) jars pureed tomatoes
- 4 cloves garlic (chopped)
- 4 (6-oz) jars tomato glue
- 1 tbsp chopped fresh basil (fresh)
- 1 tbsp chopped parsley (fresh) + extra 1 tbsp
- 2 lbs ground meat
- 1 cup dry bread pieces
- 1 lb ground pork
- 1 cup ground Parmesan cheddar

Method:

- In a big pot, blend the sliced garlic, pureed tomatoes and glue, 1 tbsp parsley, and basil.
- Heat this sauce to the point of boiling, then turn the heat down to low to stew the sauce.
- In a bowl, combine as one the pork, hamburger, bread morsels, parmesan cheddar, 1 tbsp parsley, and garlic powder.

- Combine this as one well, then structure into balls generally the size of a golf ball.
- Fry the meatballs in a skillet in hot olive oil until they are altogether cooked.
- Add the meatballs to the sauce blend and cover.
- Let it stew on low for around four hours.
- Serve over noodles of your decision.

34: Tiramisu

Perhaps the most mainstream cookies that can guarantee itself as an extraordinary top pick among everything is the Italian Tiramisu. Each café that serves Italian food makes certain to have it on its menu. Tiramisu was conceived distinctly in the 1970s in Veneto, Italy. It acquired prominence all through the world a lot later just in the mid-nineties.

This pastry contains ingredients that don't seem to mix well with one another however when used to the correct extents comes out as a lip-smacking sweet. Every one of the ingredients is so not quite the same as one another that, astonishingly, a particularly superb desert can be acquired when these ingredients are blended in the legitimate extents. Every one of these ingredients is sweet without help from anyone else.

Ingredients:

- 1/2 cup sweet Marsala wine
- 1 lb Mascarpone cheddar at room temperature

- 6 egg yolks
- 1/2 cups heated water
- 1/2 mug espresso seasoned alcohol
- 5 tsp moment espresso powder
- 12 ounces' ladyfingers or cut wipe cake
- Unsweetened cocoa (for cleaning)
- 1 cup sugar
- 1-ounce semi-sweet chocolate (ground) - optional

Method:

- In a bowl, blend 1/2 cups of heated water with the moment espresso.
- Mix until the espresso has broken up, then add the alcohol.
- Dunk in 1 ladyfinger at a time, quickly turning it to cover.
- Reduce it from the fluid and spot it on the lower part of an 8 x 8-inch dish. Line all espresso-covered ladyfingers one next to the other until a large part of the skillet's base is covered.
- Pour half of the mascarpone cheddar (or cream cheddar blend) over the highest point of the ladyfingers.
- Add another layer of covered woman fingers and cheddar.
- Refrigerate this for around 4 hours, or until the sweet is firm.
- Not long before serving, dust the top with cocoa.

- Embellish with the ground semi-sweet chocolate (whenever wanted) and slice into squares to serve.

Chapter: 4 Salad Dressing Recipes

35: Tomatoes and Sweet Onion Dressing

Tomatoes and sweet onion with Roquefort dressing is a conventional Italian salad that effectively loans itself well to Italian dinners like Osso Bucco and lighter meals, for example, salad and Minestrone.Mainstream Italian eateries, for example, Olive Garden serve comparative dinners of soup and salad.The excellence of this Italian salad is that it is flexibleto the point that it tends to be presented with pretty much any dinner.

Ingredients:

- Sweet onions
- Ready tomatoes
- Essential Italian Dressing
- Roquefort cheddar
- Green scallions
- Dried oregano
- Pepper
- Salt

Method:

- Cut ready red tomatoes and sweet onions exceptionally dainty.
- Spot four tomato cuts on each plate.
- Over the highest point of the tomatoes lay the onion cuts.
- Sprinkle super Basic Italian Dressing.

- Spot the two green scallions along the edge of the plate.
- Disintegrate the Roquefort cheddar over the top and sprinkle with dried oregano.
- Season to taste with salt and pepper.

36: Lemon Tahini Dressing

Tahini sauce is an incredibly adaptable dressing that is an ideal supplement to everything from sandwiches to rice, pasta, and even meat dishes. Yet, perhaps the best blending is with fresh vegetables, which are changed from standard to exceptional with a delightful Lemon Tahini Dressing. This lemon tahini dressing is not difficult to make this delectable. It's creamy with a tart lemon flavor and goes so well with all your favorite salads.

Ingredients:

- Black pepper to taste
- 2/3 to 3/4 cups water (depending on the situation)
- 1/2 cup tahini
- 3 tablespoons fresh lemon juice
- 1 tablespoon olive oil
- 1 clove garlic, crushed
- 3/4 teaspoon ocean salt (or to taste)

Method:

- Whisk or mix all ingredients, beginning with 2/3 cup water and adding more until you arrive at an ideal consistency.
- The dressing will hold 5 to 6 days in the fridge.

37: Super Cabbage Juice

Do your children wrinkle their noses at the name of the vegetable? Well, that isn't generally excellent information as it is vital to remember cabbage for your child's diet. This tough and solid vegetable is bountiful in dietary benefit. It is plentiful in Vitamin A, B, C, and E and ensures your eyes and skin, improves your digestion, assists with consuming fat, and is a powerful enemy of oxidant. If your kids won't eat the vegetable, you can evaluate cabbage soup recipes of various types and have confidence your children will smack their lips.

Ingredients:

- 3 carrots
- 6 green onions
- 2 green peppers
- 1 container of mushroom
- 2 jars of tomato
- A lot of celery
- 1 package of Lipton soup blend
- Half top of a cabbage
- Pepper, salt, garlic powder, parsley, and curry for preparing

Method:

- Cut the onions and utilize a cooking splash to sauté them in a pot.
- Cut the stem off the green pepper and afterward cut it into equal parts. Reduce the film and the seeds. Make bit size pieces and add to the pot.
- Reduce the leaves of the cabbage, dice it and throw it in the pot.
- Cut the carrots and celery into little pieces and add to the pot
- Cut the mushrooms thickly and add them.
- Add the tomatoes.
- Add garlic powder if you need to.
- Add 12 cups of water; cover the pot and let your soup cook for several hours.

38: Vinegar Dressing

Vinegar dressing can be alluded to as vinaigrettes. For making a vinaigrette presumably the most normal enhanced vinegar which is the white vinegar isn't the ideal sort of vinegar for making a dressing. You can use white wine vinegar. Then again, the sorts and kinds of particularly made vinegar including balsamic, raspberry, or sherry are as various and as shifted it very well maybe

Vinegar dressing has been used to enhance dishes for a ton of years at this point and is the most loved dressing utilized these days by culinary experts to improve dinner or salad that may somehow or another be boring to introduce. The ease of the vinegar is truly what keeps it normal and is broadly used even inside your family cooking.

Ingredients:

- 1 tablespoon white wine vinegar
- 3 tablespoons extra virgin olive oil
- Squeeze genuine salt
- A turn of freshly ground black pepper
- 1-2 tablespoons fresh cleaved spices
- A finely crushed garlic clove
- 2 teaspoons finely cleaved shallots, scallions, or onion
- 2 teaspoons finely crushed or ground ginger
- 2 tablespoons finely ground or disintegrated Parmesan
- 1 teaspoon Dijon mustard
- Spot of squashed red pepper chips
- 1/2 - 1 teaspoon sugar or honey

Method:

- Add the whole of the ingredients to a little bricklayer container, screw on the top, and shake until mixed.
- You can likewise whisk the ingredients together in a bowl or whirr them together in a blender.
- Taste and change flavors whenever wanted.
- Add to salad, prepare, and serve.
- Keep extra dressing in a fixed container in the fridge for 2 - 3 days.

39: Honey Raspberry Vinaigrette

Honey Raspberry Vinaigrette is a sweet recipe. It's an incredible salad dressing for the warm spring and midyear months and adds a brilliant fly of raspberry flavor to any salad recipe. This raspberry dressing is very flexible. However, I love it on my Berry Spinach Salad for an extra increase in raspberry goodness.

Basic, fresh, and modest, the flavors in this custom-made Raspberry Vinaigrette recipe are such a ton better than anything you can purchase at the store! Mix up a clump to keep in your refrigerator to add a sweet and lively kick to all your late spring salad.

Ingredients:

- 2/3 cup balsamic vinegar
- 1 cup fresh raspberries
- 1/4 cup olive oil
- 1 tablespoon white sugar
- 1 tablespoon honey
- 1/2 teaspoon salt

Method:

- Consolidate raspberries and white sugar in a bowl and leave for 10 to 15 minutes until the blend is delicious.
- Crush berries utilizing a fork until condensed (or beat in a blender for 30 seconds if you lean toward dressing to be smoother).

- Fill a glass container with a top then add balsamic vinegar, honey, olive oil, and salt to the container.
- Cover and shake until very much consolidated.

Refrigerate until prepared to utilize.

40: Messy Peppercorn Dressing

Peppercorn dressings are an extraordinary method to introduce particular and remarkable flavors to the bed while giving a sprinkle of splendid tones. A rainbow of hot flavors like white, green, and pink can without much of a stretch make a noteworthy dish. Messy Peppercorn Dressing is a brilliantly smooth dressing with a hot kick from fresh broke peppercorns! It's stunning over salad or utilized as a plunge with vegetable crudités.

Ingredient:

- 1/2 teaspoon salt, or more to taste
- 2 cups plain low-fat yogurt
- 1/4 cup finely chopped green onion
- 1/4 cup ground parmesan cheddar, or more to taste
- 2 tablespoons milk
- 1 tablespoon mayonnaise
- 2 tablespoons finely cut fresh parsley
- 2 teaspoons freshly ground black pepper

Method:

- In a bowl, combine as one yogurt, parmesan cheddar, onion, parsley mayonnaise, ground black pepper, and salt.
- Gradually add and mix in milk until wanted slenderness is accomplished.
- Add more cheddar or salt to change the taste.
- Cover and refrigerate at any rate 1 hour before serving.

41: Sweet Bacon Dressing

A straightforward salad with spinach leaves, mushrooms, and red onion gets deserving of an uncommon event when finished off with older style Sweet Bacon Dressing. So sweet and pungent with huge loads of bacon flavor and a little tang. Thoroughly long for commendable.

Ingredients:

- 1/2 cup white vinegar
- 3 teaspoons corn starch
- 1/4 cup water
- 1/2 teaspoon salt
- 1/2 cups white sugar
- 8 cuts bacon, cooked and disintegrated

Method:

- Whisk together sugar, corn starch, and salt in a medium bowl.
- Gradually mix in vinegar and water, whisking continually.
- Spot disintegrated bacon in a skillet over medium heat then pour sugar blend over bacon.
- Cook and mix continually until the combination thickens.
- Reduce from heat and permit to cool for 10 to 15 minutes before serving.

42: Creamy Cilantro Salad Dressing

This Creamy Cilantro Dressing just requires a couple of moments to make and is such a great deal better compared to locally acquired salad dressing. It is incredible on fish, mixed greens, chicken, steak, tacos, vegetables, and then some. It's really simple to make and endures a decent week in the refrigerator. It's flexible and can be utilized as a plunging sauce for veggies and fries, or as a salad dressing, on tacos or barbecued meats, burrito bowls, and on pretty much anything!

Ingredients:

- 2 cloves garlic, squashed
- 1/2 cups mayonnaise
- 2 Anaheim Chile peppers, cooked
- 1/3 cup toasted pumpkin seeds
- 3/4 cup canola oil
- 1/4 cup disintegrated Cotija cheddar
- 1/2 teaspoon salt
- 1/4 cup red wine vinegar
- 1/4 cup water
- 1/4 teaspoon freshly ground black pepper
- 2 packages cilantro, stems reduced

Method:

- Join garlic, mayonnaise, pumpkin seeds, Chile peppers, oil, water, salt, cheddar, and black pepper in a blender or food processor for 1 moment or until smooth.

- Add cilantro in groups, beating for around 40 seconds for each clump.
- Pour combination in a glass bowl.
- Cover and refrigerate for 1 hour before serving.

43: Simple Sweet and Spicy Salad Dressing

This Spicy Sweet Salad Dressing Recipe is a basic vinaigrette made with only 5 ingredients. It requires 5 minutes to make and is amazing to dress an assortment of salads. It's so totally sweet and fiery and is a simple method to light up your ordinary salad.

Ingredients:

- 1 cup vegetable oil
- 1 cup crushed onion
- 3/4 cup white sugar
- 1/4 cup apple juice vinegar
- 1/3 cup ketchup
- 1 tablespoon Worcestershire sauce

Method:

- Mix onion, ketchup, sugar, apple juice vinegar, and Worcestershire sauce in a bowl until sugar has broken down.
- Cautiously mix in vegetable oil until completely consolidated.
- Cover and refrigerate for 60 minutes.
- Mix before serving.

44: Apple and Celery Stuffing

Celery and apples share a ton for all intents and purpose; they're fresh, succulent, and delightful wellsprings of dietary fiber and vitamin C. Yet, it's the manners by which they contrast that makes them a particularly novel and free combo.

Ingredients:

- 1/2 stick of spread or margarine
- 1/2 tsp of crushed garlic (optional)
- 1 medium onion, cut fine
- 1 tsp dried sage
- 4 - 6 celery ribs, washed and cut fine
- 1 tsp dried thyme
- 1 sweet apple (any assortment) stripped, cored, and cut fine
- 1/2 cup chicken stock or stock
- around 8 ounces of dried breadcrumbs or stuffing blocks

Method:

- Dissolve the spread in a big skillet and sauté the onion and garlic over low heat until just mollified.
- Add the celery and apples; blend well and keep on sauting for a few minutes, until allingredients are covered and are starting tomollify.
- Add the breadcrumbs or stuffing 3D squares and throw them in the container to cover, then add

the stock and keep on cooking for around three minutes, or until the fluid is very much assimilated and the pieces or 3D shapes are soaked.

45: The Greek Salad

If you are searching for something luscious yet sound and wellness agreeable, go for the Greek salad unquestionably. Greek salad is a scrumptious summer dish that started in Greece. It is likewise called 'summer salad' in certain nations however locals call it horiatiki Salata, 'country salad,' or 'town salad,' which fundamental ingredients incorporate delicious tomatoes, cucumbers, green chime pepper or yellow ringer pepper, cubed feta cheddar, red onion, and Kalamata olives, with salt, dried oregano, and olive oil flavors. A few however incorporate vinegar, berries of escapades, lemon juice, and parsley to add taste.

Ingredients:
- Dried oregano - 1/2 tsp
- Ocean salt - 1/4 tsp ocean salt
- Clove garlic - 1 piece, crushed
- Extra virgin olive oil - 3 tablespoons
- Black pepper - 1/4 teaspoon
- Cucumber cut into thick parts
- Tomatoes cut into wedges
- Onion rings
- Sweet yellow pepper, in lumps
- Basil leaves (optional)

- Feta cheddar - around 120 grams, cubed
- Green ringer pepper, julienned
- Lemon juice - 1/2 tablespoons (optional)
- Kalamata olives

Method:

- To start with, you blend olive oil, garlic, lemon juice, salt, pepper, and oregano.
- Then, you blend every one of the vegetables in a single bowl and add the dressing.
- Present with black pepper to finish.

46: Tomato Mozzarella Salad

Look at this extraordinary-looking and incredible tasting dish! Since this tomato mozzarella salad has red tomatoes, white mozzarella, and green basil, the tones look extraordinary together, and the dish tastes incredible as well. The blend of fresh mozzarella cheddar, red tomatoes, and green basil makes this dish extraordinary to take a gander at, and it makes the salad scrumptious! Besides, when you are adding a spice like basil, which adds a green tone, you will make the salad much more delicious and surprisingly more beautiful.

This tomato salad is not difficult to make. Simply consolidate chopped tomatoes, fresh mozzarella cheddar, and basil. Utilize a touch of olive oil and balsamic vinegar to gently dress this salad. Or then again, avoid the vinegar and simply utilize olive oil to dress it - it will in any case be exceptionally delectable.

Ingredients:

- 1/2 little white onion, cubed little
- 3 cups sweet grape, cherry, or bigger cleaved tomatoes
- 2/3 cup little cubed mozzarella cheddar
- 2/3 tablespoon balsamic vinegar (great quality)
- 1 tablespoon extra-virgin olive oil (great quality)
- 4 leaves of romaine lettuce (measured to suit the size of servings you need)
- Italian parsley for decorate
- Salt and pepper to taste

Method:

- Blend the above ingredients in a bowl.
- Mix the olive oil and vinegar in a cup by beating them along with a fork.
- Blend this in well with the tomato combination.
- Season the blend with pepper and salt (according to taste).
- Spoon the tomato combination into an appealing heap on top of the lettuce and trimming with parsley.
- Serve this immediately...you don't need your lettuce to get unstable.
- Enjoy!

47: Cobb Salad

This is quite possibly the most loved salad arrangement of people across the world. With every one of the ingredients like eggs, bacon, chickens, and salad dressing, it simply tastes marvelous! Go through this basic recipe given underneath. It requires just 50 minutes to finish and serve the salad at your table.

Ingredients:

- Three eggs
- 8 cuts of bacon
- 1 head destroyed ice shelf lettuce
- Two cultivated and cut tomatoes
- 3 cups chicken meat (cut, cooked)
- disintegrated blue cheddar - 3/4 cup
- 1 stripped, pitted, and cubed avocado
- Farm style salad dressing - 1 (8 ounce) bottle
- 3 chopped green onions

Method:

- Put eggs in a skillet and with cold water cover the eggs.
- Allow the water to bubble. Put a cover, reduce it from heat, and let the eggs stay in the hot water for around 10 to 12 minutes.
- Take the eggs out from the boiling water, cool them down, strip and afterward hack them.
- Spot the cuts of bacon in a major, profound skillet.

- Cook the bacon cuts on medium-high heat until every one of the cuts is consistently earthy colored on all sides.
- Strain, disintegrate the pieces, and put away the pieces.
- Separate the destroyed lettuce in the various plates similarly.
- Similarly gap and spot bacon, chicken, tomatoes, blue cheddar, eggs, green onions, and avocado in a line on top of the chunk of ice lettuce leaves.
- Sprinkle with Ranch-style salad dressing as per your necessities and enjoy the salad.
- You can utilize feta cheddar rather than blue cheddar.
- You can embellish it with cheddar and bubbled corn.
- You can add vegetables like carrots, zucchini, yellow squash, cabbages, and so forth to make it nutritious.
- You can likewise add mayonnaise if you need to make a rich surface.
- You can likewise utilize serve this salad with singed chicken wings.

48: Shrimp and Avocado Salad

This is a stunning salad recipe that is incredible as a side salad or as a light lunch meeting recipe. Serve it in lettuce cups for lunch alongside some fresh hard bread and an extraordinary treat. Simply awesome!

Ingredients:

- 1 avocado
- 1 cup celery, meagerly cut
- 2 tablespoons Italian salad dressing
- salt and pepper to taste
- 4 tablespoons mayonnaise
- 2 teaspoons lemon juice
- 1 pound frozen cooked shrimp, defrosted

Method:

- Join the shrimp, celery, Italian dressing, and mayonnaise.
- Season to taste with salt and pepper.
- Chill, covered until prepared to serve.
- When prepared to serve, strip and dice the avocado.
- Blend promptly with the lemon juice to keep the avocado from going dull.
- Add to the shrimp combination and blend delicately.

49: Cucumber Salad

This recipe is scrumptious, however quite simple. It's an extraordinary recipe to serve the organization at a grill since it stretches made beyond and sits in the cooler for a couple of hours until you are prepared for it. The best summer engaging plans do not need the host and entertainer to be in the kitchen cooking while visitors relax outside.

Ingredients:

- 1/4 cups red wine vinegar
- 3 huge cucumbers, stripped and meagerly cut
- 1/2 teaspoon celery salt
- 1 tablespoon honey
- 1/2 head of lettuce, destroyed
- a great squeeze of black pepper
- 4 tablespoons olive oil
- 1/2 teaspoon fresh dill, cleaved
- 1 teaspoon Dijon mustard

Method:

- Prepare every one of the ingredients completely in a huge salad bowl.
- Chill for 2 hours before serving.

50: Lime Jello Cottage Cheese Salad

This is an exquisite light salad recipe that is ideal for a late spring grill yet functions admirably throughout the year on a smorgasbord table. The expansion of curds may sound odd; however, it is an extraordinary flavor that blends in with the Jello. The mash of the celery and green pepper add another layer of flavor and fresh taste.

Ingredients:

- 1 cup bubbling water
- 1 - 3-ounce package lime jam powder
- 1/2 cup cold water
- 1/2 cup mayonnaise

- salt and pepper
- 1 teaspoon vinegar or lemon juice
- 3/4 cup cleaved celery
- 1/2 green pepper, cleaved
- 1/2 onion, cleaved

Method:

- Mix with mixer and chill until firm 1" from the edge of the dish.
- Transform it into a bowl and beat it until it turns out to be light and fleecy.
- Overlap in 1 cup curds, celery, onion, and green pepper.
- Chill completely before serving.

51: Pork Chops

Searching for various approaches to fix pork hacks? Eating them seared is delectable and filling however there are numerous alternative ways that they can be readied that will draw out the very scrumptious flavor that you love. Attempt Pork Chops basic and delectable recipe for a scrumptious option in contrast to ordinary searing. Pork hacks can be utilized to make astonishing meals that too consistently. These are the simplest dishes that one can make at home. The plans for pork slashes are not muddled and fabulous plans can be made with them.

Ingredients:

- 1/3 cup bourbon

- 1 tsp black pepper
- 1/3 cup soy sauce (low sodium)
- 2 tbsp. juice vinegar
- 3 cloves garlic
- 3 tbsp. Brown sugar
- 1 tsp red pepper pieces
- 1 tbsp. cornstarch

Method:

- Combine the initial seven ingredients as one.
- Save ¼ cup of the blend.
- Pour the leftover marinade over the pork hacks in a fixed plastic sack.
- Refrigerate the pork hacks for the time being.
- Before flame broiling the cleaves, blend cornstarch into the ¼ cup of unused marinade.
- Tenderly heat until effervescent and thickened into a brilliant sauce.
- Serve the grilled pork cleaves with a spoonful of the sauce over the top.

52: Hot Green Bean Salad with Potatoes

Bean salad is consistently a success at summer grills and family social affairs. They are not difficult to plan, modest to make, and make an extraordinary backup to any feast. Attempt this Hot Green Bean Salad with Potatoes recipe at your next family gathering. Your family will make certain to adore it.

Ingredients:

- 2 tbsp. olive oil
- 1 cut onion finely cut
- 1 little or ½ medium onion, chopped
- 1/8 tsp salt
- 2 tbsp. corn starch
- 1/8 tsp black pepper
- 1 to 1 ¼ cup sugar
- 1 cup white vinegar
- 2 to 4 medium potatoes, cubed and cooked
- 32 oz. Green beans, cooked
- 4 cuts of bacon, disintegrated

Method:

- Cut bacon into little pieces with kitchen shears.
- Fry the bacon until firm.
- Spot the bacon on a paper towel to deplete the bacon fat.
- In a spotless profound fry, the dish adds olive oil, little cleaved onion, salt, and pepper.
- Cook over medium heat until the onion has a marginally brilliant shading.
- Keep cooking the onion and add the corn starch and blend into the onion completely.
- Add the sugar and blend once more.
- Add the vinegar to the whole blend and continue to mix over the heat until every one of the ingredients has merged.
- Permit the combination to cook until hot and effervescent. When the sauce has thickened, reduce the heat.
- Cook the green beans and potatoes together until both are delicate.
- Flush and channel in a colander.
- Spot the beans and potatoes into a serving dish.
- Pour the warm sauce on the potatoes & beans.
- Sprinkle the finely cleaved onion on top alongside the firm bacon bits.

53: Spinach and Cranberry Salad

Spinach and Cranberry Salad are wonderful! It's a fast and simple salad you can gather in around ten to fifteen minutes. What's more, that incorporates making the dressing! It just uses a modest bunch of ingredients making the simplicity of planning extremely basic. This delicious salad incorporates spinach, red onion, goat cheddar, almonds, and dried cranberries.

Ingredients:

- 1 cup dried cranberries
- 1 lb. spinach, flushed and attacked pieces
- 2 tbsp. crushed onion
- 1 tbsp. margarine
- 3/4 cup almonds, whitened and fragmented
- 2 tbsp. toasted sesame seeds
- 1/4 tbsp. paprika
- 1 tbsp. poppy seeds
- 1/2 cup white sugar
- 1/4 cup white wine vinegar
- 1/2 cup vegetable oil
- 1/4 cup juice vinegar

Method:

- Heat a little skillet at medium heat and liquefy the margarine.
- Add the almonds and cook until toasted. Permit the almonds to cool.

- In a huge bowl, combine as one the cranberries, spinach, and almonds.
- In a different bowl, whisk together the sugar, vegetable oil, white wine vinegar, juice vinegar, onion, poppy seeds, paprika, and sesame seeds.
- Not long before serving, throw the spinach in the dressing blend.

54: Broccoli Salad with a Twist

Most Broccoli Salads have Mayonnaise as the essential ingredient. However, this Salad utilizes Cream Cheese which adds a decent flavor and the apple juice gives it a truly fun zip. Likewise, the calorie distinction is insane. For the Mayonnaise salad, there are around 1495 calories. This Easy Salad utilizes Cream Cheese, which slices the calories to 776!!!! Fundamentally, for 6 servings this salad (without the bacon!) is 129 calories for each serving contrasted with 250 calories for the mayonnaise.

Ingredients:

- 1/3 cup mandarin oranges
- 3 tbsp. mayonnaise
- 1/2 cups fresh broccoli florets
- 4 bacon strips, cooked and chopped
- 1/4 cup finely cleaved onion
- 1 tbsp. sugar
- 3/4 cup destroyed cheddar
- 2 tbsp. white vinegar

Method:

- In a big bowl combine as one the broccoli, bacon, onion, and cheddar.
- In a different bowl, join the mayo, sugar, and vinegar-blend well.
- Pour the sauce over the broccoli combination and combine as one.
- Cover with saran wrap and refrigerate for at least 60 minutes.
- Not long before serving, sprinkle chilled mandarin oranges over the top.

55: Pear and Pecan Salad

Simple to prepare ahead, this spinach salad is loaded up with sweet cooked pears, smooth walnuts, tart goat cheddar, crunchy pomegranates with a simple hand-crafted balsamic dressing is an ideal occasion side dish or a scrumptious fall meal. This Roasted Pear Salad is a recipe you will be eager to set aside a few minutes and time once more.

Ingredients:

- 1/3 cup Italian salad dressing
- 1 pack Italian salad
- 1/2 cup walnut parts
- 1/2 cup destroyed mozzarella cheddar
- 1 pear (stripped, cored, and cubed)

Method:

- Throw all ingredients (aside from dressing) in a bowl.
- When prepared to serve, sprinkle a touch of Italian dressing over the blend and throw well to guarantee an in any event, covering.
- Topping with lemon or mandarin oranges.

56: Pistachio Fruit Salad

Making this pistachio salad is speedy, simple, and modest. It doesn't make any difference if you call it Watergate salad, pistachio cushion, or pistachio fruit salad, they're all names for a similar delightful pastry. Any gathering is an incredible chance to prepare a cluster of this pistachio salad. I realize I continue to call this a salad when it is more similar to a sweet.

Ingredients:

- 1 package moment without sugar pistachio pudding blend
- 1 cup decreased fat whipped besting
- 1 can fruit mixed drink, depleted
- 1 can mandarin oranges, depleted
- 1/4 cup maraschino cherries
- 1 can squashed pineapple
- A modest bunch of small scale marshmallows

Method:

- Channel the pineapple juice into a huge bowl.
- Rush in the pudding blend for around two minutes.

- Add pineapple, fruit mixed drink, oranges, cherries, and marshmallows.
- Cautiously crease in the whipped garnish to keep it fleecy.
- Cover with saran wrap and refrigerate until serving.

Chapter: 5 Ginger Recipes

57: Ginger Pesto Chicken

Figure out how to cook extraordinary Chicken with ginger pesto. Crecipe.com conveys the fine determination of value Chicken with ginger pestoplans furnished with appraisals, audits, and blending tips. Get one of our Chicken with ginger pesto recipesand plan a delightful and solid treat for your family or companions. Great hunger.

Ingredients:

- 2 cloves garlic, crushed
- 1 kg. boneless and skinless chicken bosom parts
- 1 pack green onions, cut into 1/4-inch pieces
- 1/4 cup vegetable oil
- 1/2 cup dry white wine
- 2 tablespoons ground fresh ginger root
- 1 teaspoon white sugar
- 1 tablespoon salt

Method:

- In a medium pot, pour 2-3 cups of softly salted water then add chicken bosoms.
- Heat to the point of boiling, lower heat, and stew for 8-10 minutes or until cooked through.
- Permit chicken to cool in the stock.
- When cool, reduce from stock and put away.

- Heat vegetable oil in a different skillet over medium-high heat then mix in garlic, ginger, salt, and sugar.
- Lower heat and cook for 15-20 minutes or until garlic is delicate.
- Mix in onions and cook for 10 minutes more until onions are delicate.
- Cut chicken bosoms daintily, orchestrate on a plate then top with the ginger combination.

58: Ginger-Glazed Salmon

A marginally sweet, yet zesty and unimaginably tasty ginger coat makes this overpowering salmon recipe that is easy to get ready and meets up in a short time. This recipe is easy to make, yet great. The marinade gives the fish a sweet taste that my family goes crazy for! If it's excessively cold out to barbecue it, you likewise may cook it. Get the flakey salmon surface you've generally needed with a delightful maple ginger sauce for sure.

Ingredients:

- 1 tablespoon Dijon mustard
- 1/2 kg. salmon filets
- 1 tablespoon honey
- 2 teaspoons olive oil
- 2 teaspoons ground fresh ginger

Method:

- Join Dijon mustard, honey, ginger, and olive oil in a little bowl.
- Spot salmon filets in a preparing dish and equally brush with the blend.
- Prepare in a pre-warmed broiler (350 degrees F) for 15-20 minutes.

59: Honey Ginger Salad Dressing

Most food sources taste better when blended in with the appropriate enhancing or dressing. Be it a fundamental dish or, a canapé, nothing beats a decent food with a similarly decent dressing. A common steak gets professional when presented with a flavorsome sauce. Fruits like strawberry work better with plunges like whipped cream or chocolate.

Make a cluster of this toward the end of the week and enjoy fresh salads throughout the week (truly, simply toss this on some child spinach, and the writing is on the wall! A salad!), or utilize some as a marinade for grilled chicken or veggies. It will remain fresh in the refrigerator for a month, leaving you a lot of time to go through it.

Ingredients:

- 3 cloves garlic, crushed
- 1 lemon, squeezed
- 1 cup olive oil
- Ground black pepper to taste
- 3 tablespoons crushed fresh ginger root

- 1/4 cup soy sauce
- 2 teaspoons honey
- 1 teaspoon arranged mustard (Dijon-style)

Method:

- Combine as one lemon juice, ginger, garlic, honey, mustard, and black pepper in a medium bowl until altogether consolidated.
- Mix in olive oil gradually and blend until joined with different ingredients.

Store in a glass compartment and refrigerate until prepared for serving.

60: Tropical Ginger Shrimp

This Tropical Ginger Shrimp finished off with shrimp and a fruit salsa is a finished meal. Big bits of ginger-soy marinated shrimp and tropical fruit salsa with mango, pineapple, kiwifruit, and mandarin oranges are delicately thrown with child spinach leaves and long strands of pasta in this tropical-enlivened dish.

Ingredients:

- Sticks
- 1 onion, cut
- 1/4 kind sized shrimp, stripped and deveined
- 2 cloves garlic, stripped
- 1/4 cup lemon juice
- 1/2 cup olive oil
- 2 tablespoons ground fresh ginger root

- 2 tablespoons crushed cilantro leaves
- 1 teaspoon paprika
- 1/2 teaspoon salt
- 2 teaspoons sesame oil
- 1/2 teaspoon ground black pepper

Method:

- Consolidate onion, lemon juice, garlic, olive oil, ginger, sesame oil, cilantro, paprika, salt, and pepper in a blender and puree until smooth.
- Save a limited quantity for treating.
- Pour the combination into a big bowl and add shrimp.
- Coat shrimp with blend, cover, and refrigerate for at any rate 2 hours.
- When prepared, dispose of abundance marinade and string shrimp onto sticks.
- Cook in a pre-warmed flame broil over medium-high heat for 2 minutes for every side or until shrimp is cooked through.
- Brush with marinade while cooking.

Conclusion:

Fasting is an extraordinary method to keep the body and psyche solid and clean. Numerous people that training Intermittent fasting consistently guarantee they've taken in a ton about their dietary patterns also. The explanation is because they have a great deal of time to consider food and which food sources they're wanting on their fasting days.

The degree of adrenaline your body produces is likewise expanded during momentary fasting, which places your body's capacity to consume fat into overdrive and work twice as hard. Join this with your expanded digestion and you can perceive how shedding pounds would be so basic with Intermittent fasting.

Intermittent fasting isn't prudent for all people. This is just useful for people without medical issues. Whenever you want to try intermittent fasting, you should counsel first with your doctor before you push through.

www.ingramcontent.com/pod-product-compliance
Lightning Source LLC
Chambersburg PA
CBHW060305030426
42336CB00011B/953